Women's Qigong

for Health and Longevity

Women's Qigong

for Health and Longevity

A PRACTICAL GUIDE
FOR WOMEN FORTY AND OVER

DEBORAH DAVIS, LAc, MAOM

SHAMBHALA

BOSTON & LONDON 2008

SHAMBHALA PUBLICATIONS, INC.
Horticultural Hall
300 Massachusetts Avenue
Boston, Massachusetts 02115
www.shambhala.com

9 8 7 6 5 4 3 2 1

First Edition

BOOK DESIGN BY DCDESIGN
PHOTOGRAPHS BY ROBERT FROST

Printed in the United States of America

⊗ This edition is printed on acid-free paper that meets the
American National Standards Institute z39.48 Standard.
Distributed in the United States by Random House, Inc.,
and in Canada by Random House of Canada Ltd.
Library of Congress Cataloging-in-Publication Data

Davis, Deborah (Deborah Atkinson), 1954–
Women's Qigong for health and longevity: a practical guide for women
forty and over, Deborah Davis.—1st ed.
p.   cm.
Includes bibliographical references.
ISBN 978-1-59030-537-9 (pbk.: alk. paper)
1. Qi gong. 2. Middle-aged women—Health and hygiene. I.Title

RA781.8.D38 2008
613.7'14082—dc22
2007048870

In loving memory of my mother,
   Who taught me the importance of beauty and laughter in life,
      and
To Ren, the guiding spirit behind this book,
   Big Qi hugs!

CONTENTS

PART THREE
Self-Healing for Women

Women's Qigong

for Health and Longevity

Introduction

THE MOST POWERFUL TOOL for healing lies within you—your breath.

Breath is our inherent gift at birth that anyone can learn to cultivate for vibrant health or remarkable healing. Can you imagine leading a dynamic life into your golden years without medication and expensive medical bills? It's as simple as a fifteen-minute daily practice of breathing exercises called Qigong, which are renowned in China for health and longevity. Our body instinctively knows how to repair itself (such as recovering from the common cold or healing abrasions), so why shouldn't we be able to enhance this natural process and consciously heal other, more serious illnesses? Western medicine has taught us to believe that self-healing is beyond our grasp, yet Chinese medicine is founded on the principle of harnessing and regulating our internal energies for the purpose of healing ourselves.

For the past few decades, Westerners have turned toward the East to glean ancient wisdom, especially concerning health care and spirituality, and Qigong is emerging as one of the hidden jewels of immortality and self-healing. These versatile exercises combine three elements—focused breathing, posture or movement, and mental concentration—to harmonize the body, mind, and spirit. "Qi" refers to life force energies and "gong" means to work or cultivate. Thus, Qigong is the practice of developing your own inner strength and vitality for optimum health.

Medical Qigong (presented in this book) is both curative and preventive. It will activate your body's Qi through the practice of slow movements and stretches, held stances, intonation of healing sounds to detoxify your organs, and self-massage on acupressure points. This low-impact exercise (very similar to tai chi) is a blend of dancelike movements and meditation, and is both relaxing and invigorating. Qigong has numerous health benefits, such as stress reduction and lowering blood pressure, without risk of injury. The movements are easy to learn, less strenuous than yoga or Pilates, and more accessible to women of varying ages and fitness levels.

Women's Qigong for Health and Vitality will enable you to care for your own well-being and heal common complaints such as hot flashes, PMS, heart problems, insomnia, and osteoporosis. By incorporating simple routines into your day, you will reclaim your vitality and emotional equilibrium, as well as increase your energy reserves, slow aging, regulate those wayward hormones, and relieve tension.

OUR POTENTIAL

According to numerous ancient Chinese texts, the human life span is 150 to 200 years, but today only a minority of people live to become centenarians. Although the life expectancy in the West has risen, our quality of life is burdened by poor diet, stress, and our preoccupation with incessant busyness. We have become divorced from our natural body rhythms and are unaware of the reservoir of energies that lies untapped within us. For over two thousand years, the Chinese have been accessing these powerful resources, and Qigong is one of the most ancient healing modalities founded on this concept of energy management.

There are many accounts of Chinese Qigong masters who have learned to use their energy to dissolve cancerous tumors with a wave of their hand, heal patients long-distance with focused intention, or make their body so weightless that they can stand on suspended rice paper without falling through! These miraculous and mysterious abilities are accomplished by disciplined Qigong training that enables them to control both their mind and body. The good news is that you don't have to be a Qigong master to experience the innumerable benefits of this ancient healing art.

MIND-BODY

The mind-body connection is a central component in Qigong. Most of us are familiar with the expression "mind over matter," like tapping into extra energy to run the last mile of a race (or those rare instances where people have been able to perform amazing feats to rescue someone in danger). The basic tenet of Qigong is that our mind and body are not separate, and focusing our mind through concentrated effort can change our internal environment. Qi can be induced and directed to a certain area or along defined routes inside our body for healing or for incredible displays of Qi power. Everyone has the potential to develop and channel their Qi. Qigong will teach you how to enhance your life force energy to experience renewal in all levels of your life. As a practitioner you can preserve organ functioning, regulate your metabolism and heart rate, and look younger as you age. You will learn to control your body and become fit from the inside out.

QIGONG AND WOMEN

Much of the Chinese Qigong history revolves around men; however, many women were also proficient at Qigong, especially as healers. Ancient female shamans and Taoist (Daoist) adepts were Qigong masters who were sought after for their remarkable abilities in divination, healing, spiritual teachings, and mastery of the body. They were able to "slay the red dragon," (i.e., stop their menstrual cycles) to redirect their energies for higher spiritual purposes. I met a Taoist nun in China who did this successfully through her Qigong practice, and she was extremely vibrant and soulful. When I asked her for one exercise that she'd recommend women practice daily, she taught me a visualization similar to the *Ren Chong* Meditation (see chapter 6, Meditations, p. 36), stating she felt it would be particularly calming and supportive for modern women.

The reemergence of Qigong's ancient healing methods is particularly relevant for women, since Western medicine has no protocols for maintaining agility and grace as we age. Women go to doctors twice as frequently as men, yet many of their complaints are not "curable" according to allopathic medicine. Conditions such as PMS, menopause, depression, fibromyalgia, and fatigue are most often controlled by pharmaceuticals, but studies now reveal that many of the standard drugs for these imbalances (such as Premarin for menopause) are fraught with deleterious side effects. The Institute for Alternative Futures reported that stress is the contributing factor for 60 to 90 percent of the medical problems confronted by physicians, problems that mind-body therapies, such as Qigong, could easily eliminate without resorting to invasive interventions.

MY APPRENTICESHIP

During my schooling in Oriental medicine, I apprenticed with Dr. Wu, a Qigong master (not his real name since he prefers to remain anonymous). As part of my apprenticeship, Dr. Wu and I ran a Qigong clinic in the early 1990s in Santa Barbara, California. While there I witnessed infertile women become pregnant, cysts disappear, chronic fatigue and clinical depression resolve, and even terminally ill cancer patients go into remission. Many women came seeking an alternative approach—the medicine of Qigong—as their last hope.

Dr. Wu taught me how to assess patients as soon as they walked in the door simply by watching how they moved, noting their speech, and observing their facial expressions. He'd listen with great care to their stories while silently weaving together a diagnosis of their mental, emotional, physical, and spiritual needs. Utilizing his training in Western and traditional Chinese medicine, he diagnosed and healed conditions that other allopathic doctors couldn't treat or had deemed incurable.

Early in my apprenticeship I was personally touched to discover that these deceptively easy exercises can have profound healing effects. When my seventy-five-year-old mother had dangerously high blood pressure that wouldn't respond to medication, I designed a Qigong protocol to lower her pressure and regulate her heart. Within a month she had the lowest pressure since her twenties. (See chapter 19, Heart Health, p. 140 for the protocol.) In another instance, a woman came to us after two years of trying all of the Western methods to treat infertility. Using a Chinese medical diagnosis, we concluded that her suppressed anger contributed to the stagnation and blockage of energy through her pelvis and reproductive organs. We prescribed Qigong exercises to express the anger out of her body and meditations to calm her anxiety. As you can imagine, she was quite frustrated that conceiving a baby had become such a project! As the weeks passed she looked healthier and experienced increased energy, joy, and a deeper capacity to handle stress in a positive way. Within six months, she became pregnant and is now the mother of three healthy children.

Although there were many times when Dr. Wu "cured" me and others, his primary message (and the guiding principle of medical Qigong) has always been the importance of taking care of oneself and learning the disciplines of self-healing. The word "heal" means to make whole, and I often remind my patients that healing is a process and not an event. By practicing the routines in this book, you will become more intimate with the nuances of your body and learn to gauge where and when you're out of balance, even before it manifests as illness.

Qigong is a profound yet gentle healing art that will activate your innate physical, mental, and spiritual powers. I've witnessed the transformation of many women through Qigong and I hope this book will inspire you into a renewed commitment to self-care. Imagine if we mobilized and expanded our vast potential to put the rest of these untapped resources to use! We would definitely experience more vital, enriched, and extended lives and come to know true harmony within ourselves.

The Root
of Qigong

1

Making Qigong a Part of Your Life

A journey of a thousand miles begins with a single step.

—Lao-tzu

Oᴜʀ ʙᴏᴅʏ ʜᴀs the miraculous capacity to mend itself and Qigong reawakens the natural healer within each of us. Through the past decade of prescribing Qigong for women's health, I've simplified the programs and have included the most successful protocols in this book. A devoted practice of fifteen to thirty minutes a day will enable you to experience increased vigor, strength, and inner calm.

The basic concepts of medical Qigong are very different than our Western approach to health and fitness. The Chinese perspective is based on prevention of disease instead of intervention. You must aspire to attain an active involvement in your health instead of passive compliance, an attitude that prevails in the allopathic approach. Active participation means that you do it for and by yourself—not that you practice solo, but that you, and you alone, are responsible for your health.

By following a consistent Qigong program, it is no longer necessary to run to a doctor every time you feel ill. Practicing Qigong will empower you to heal yourself and your family—it is an inner resource, one that is free, abundant, and available to anyone who desires to increase her energy and personal serenity.

HOW TO USE THIS BOOK

Part 1: The Root of Qigong

This section introduces the basic concepts of Chinese medicine and Qigong healing. It includes a chapter describing how you can explore your own Qi field and energetic boundaries. Subsequent chapters introduce Qigong breathing, warm-up exercises, stances, and meditations, all of which will become a part of your daily routine. I recommend that you begin by learning the basic *dantian* breathing until this deep abdominal respiration feels comfortable to you. This is an important prerequisite since proper technique insures success with all of the exercises outlined in the book.

Chapter 7, Five-Element Healing, delves into the philosophy of Chinese medical thought and offers suggestions to deepen your connection to these elements in Nature. The Six Healing Sounds (chapter 8) are referred to in most routines, but this series can also be done as a separate practice to regulate the organs and balance your emotions. (You can learn these exercises and hear the sounds corresponding to each of the organs on my DVD, *The Spirit of Qi Gong: Chinese Exercises for Longevity*. Ordering information is on page 163.)

Part 2: Healthy, Fit, and Sexy at Any Age

This portion of the book features Qigong programs that will enable you to remain healthy, fit, and sexy throughout your life. The age delineations are loosely based on the traditional Chinese theory that major shifts in a woman's life occur every seven years (eight for men). Since women have different concerns and health issues as they age, it is important to have Qigong routines that address these changes. A forty-year-old woman needs a more vital and challenging program than a woman in her seventies. Follow the program recommended for your age group and add supplementary exercises to fit your personal needs. For instance, if you're going through perimenopause in your early forties, then practice the exercises outlined in chapter 10, Graceful Passage, along with a few exercises from chapter 9, Dynamic Woman. In addition, if you have a particular health challenge described in part 3, Self-Healing for Women, then adopt the relevant protocol for your daily practice or include those exercises in your age-related workout.

For easy reference, the Appendix contains all of the Qigong programs described in this book, listing the routines for each age group and imbalance.

Part 3: Self-Healing for Women

This section is composed of chapters that cover the most prevalent issues for women forty and older that I see in my clinic: PMS, depression, breast health, menopause, heart problems/hypertension, insomnia, breast cancer, osteoporosis, and low sexual vitality. If you are facing a health challenge, simply turn to the chapter that best describes your condition and perform that sequence daily. Or if you have a genetic predisposition for a particular illness but have not manifested any symptoms, I recommend following the exercises for that ailment two to three times a week as a preventive measure, along with your age-specific Qigong. For example, if anyone in your family has had breast cancer, do the breast exercises three times a week to maintain healthy tissue and keep the flow of beneficial Qi in the chest.

Each chapter contains a comprehensive Qigong plan, along with contemplations to deepen your emotional healing. It features discussions of basic Chinese medical theory in relation to Qigong are accompanied with stories of women who have healed themselves through these programs.

The Qigong routines are outlined in a four-step process to create a complete healing program:

1. Dynamic Exercises to move Qi and direct healing to select organ/meridian systems;
2. Stances to build immunity and strength;
3. Self-Healing Massage to relax and move blockages; and
4. Meditation to calm the mind and emotions.

Begin your practice by focusing your mind on *dantian* breathing. This settles your thoughts and creates a quiet inner space to do your Qigong practice. One of the main differences between Qigong and other exercises is that you center your attention inward on your Qi, instead of listening to music or reading, which is a common practice on the gym machines. This is a mind-body practice that combines concentration and relaxation. For best results practice half an hour once or twice a day. If you're seeking healing from cancer or a chronic illness then one to two hours a day (or more) is optimal for a faster recovery.

FREQUENTLY ASKED QUESTIONS ABOUT QIGONG PRACTICE

Can anyone do Qigong?

Qigong can be performed by anyone. When I was in China, I witnessed people of all ages, particularly seniors, begin their day with Qigong exercises in the parks. I have taught Qigong to women of various age and fitness levels—from triathletes to a ninety-two-year-old woman, as well as children, cancer patients and bedridden clients. This book is designed for women in their early forties through their post-menopausal years. The exercises are easy to perform and will not strain the body if done properly. By incorporating Qigong into your day, you will stay healthy, vital, and centered no matter how old you are.

How soon will I see results?

Most people feel the effects of Qigong immediately. My students report that the deep abdominal breathing alone gives them an increased sense of relaxation and an ability to handle stress more effectively. As I perform Qigong I feel a deep inner peace and spiritual connection within myself. Each morning has become a moving meditation and this tranquility remains with me throughout the day. The exercises are simple to learn and can be done anywhere—at home, in the office, or out in the serenity of Nature.

What should I wear?

Aim for function, rather than fashion! You want to be comfortable, so wear loose-fitting clothing, especially around your waist. Blue jeans are too tight and restrict the flow of Qi. Breathable material like cotton is best. I prefer to go barefoot so I can have a more intimate connection with the Earth's energy. If you need more support or if the ground is wet or cold, then I recommend that you wear sneakers. No high heels or platform shoes!

When should I practice?

The best time to practice Qigong is when you first wake up, when the air is still and quiet. This will set the tone and keep you focused and energized throughout your day. Wait for at least an hour after eating before doing Qigong, since you don't want to interfere with digestion. I usually have a protein drink or toast in the morning to keep my blood sugar stable while I do my practice and then eat afterward. If your tendency is to reach for snacks or caffeine in the afternoon, this would be another good time to practice Qigong (instead of downing lattes or energy drinks to catch a second wind). If insomnia is one of your issues, then I suggest performing the Six Healing Sounds before going to bed. However, I wouldn't recommend doing any of the other Qigong exercises at night as they can be too energizing.

Where should I practice?

I prefer to be outdoors near trees or water, away from noise and other distractions. I usually find a quiet spot on the beach, in the woods, or in our town park where I can be still and inward during my practice. If you live in the city, go to an arboretum or local park, or stay at home as long as you remember to turn off the phone, music, and TV. Qigong is meditation in movement, so it is important to have a quiet environment, free of stimuli, where the mind can be at peace. Be sure to exercise where the air is clean (without exhaust), since you will be oxygenating your body with the Qi in your environment. The Chinese believe that mountaintops infused with the healing energy of pine trees and evergreens have the most Qi, especially if they are sacred mountains.

How long should I practice?

The optimal amount of time is at least thirty minutes (or more) a day. Some of you will practice diligently while others may eke out only fifteen minutes a few times a week—even this short amount of time is beneficial. Do the best you can. If you have a chronic or terminal illness, then thirty to sixty minutes (or more) twice a day is recommended. To insure success, examine your schedule and personal habits and create a positive routine that you know you'll follow. Consistency is the key, even if it's a few minutes a day. Commit to self-healing.

Are there any precautions?

Don't do Qigong if you have an acute inflammation, fever, or internal bleeding, or during menstruation if you bleed heavily (Qigong increases your blood flow). Please consult a health practitioner before starting a new exercise program, especially if you have serious health issues or if you're pregnant. (Special note: If you're trying to build up your energy, especially with a chronic condition, then don't have sex after your Qigong practice. This will dissipate the Qi you have just cultivated instead of using it to build immunity and strength.)

What are the components of a typical routine?

- *Dantian* breathing practice (until this becomes second nature).
- Warm-up exercises.
- Qigong exercise routine—a combination of exercises for your age group, along with those you may add if you have a particular health concern.
- Stance—this can be done before or after your Qigong exercises.

- Massage—this can be done anytime during the day or in bed upon awaking or retiring. If you have a specific health concern, be sure to follow the recommendations outlined in the relevant chapters.
- Meditation—most women find morning meditation helps to focus their intentions for the day, while an evening sit assists in settling the mind for a more peaceful rest.

You can exercise by yourself, form a practice group with friends, or share the routine with your family. You may also consult your acupuncturist to determine which meridian/organ systems to add to the program you choose. More than just a gentle exercise program, Qigong will become a way of life. Enjoy your new exploration of Qi!

2

The Energetic Body

UNDERSTANDING CHINESE MEDICINE AND MEDICAL QIGONG

Everyone has a doctor in him or her;
we just have to help it in its work.

—HIPPOCRATES

QIGONG COMPRISES ANCIENT healing exercises that have been documented for over two thousand years. Today millions of Chinese practice this discipline to maintain their health and agility, and it has become the cornerstone of preventive health for China's burgeoning population. Due to its resurgence in popularity, hospitals and clinics incorporate medical Qigong with acupuncture, herbal remedies, and allopathic medicine for a holistic approach to healing. There are even specialty clinics that use solely Qigong for conditions ranging from heart disease to terminal illnesses. Patients, some who were carried in on stretch-ers, learn and practice these healing exercises, sometimes for hours throughout the day. And once cured, many of these "terminally ill" people will stay on to teach, sharing their extraordinary healing journeys with others.

Various schools of Qigong (in addition to hundreds of individual exercises) have migrated to the West: (1) martial arts Qigong; (2) Taoist Qigong; (3) Buddhist Qigong; and (4) medical Qigong. Martial arts Qigong is the most popular in China, emphasizing dynamic exercise to increase inner power and force—the hallmark of a superior fighter. The Shaolin Temple monks are famous for displaying an almost supernatural strength and agility as a result of developing command of their inner Qi.

The Taoist and Buddhist Qigong forms, illuminate their respective philosophies: both are more meditative, focusing on spiritual clarity and peace of mind. Taoist Qigong reflects the human interdependence with Nature and the Universe and includes *mudras* (meditative hand positions), sound healing, and sexual Qigong, similar to tantra. The Buddhist school seeks to cultivate a clear mind, free of distractions, with the intention to develop wisdom and compassion. In order to empower practitioners to achieve this heightened consciousness, Qigong prepares the body to become peaceful and strong, so the mind has a sound place to rest.

Medical Qigong is used for the prevention and healing of disease and imbalances. It incorporates principles and exercises from the other schools of Qigong and is composed of an internal and external form. The internal method is the most important step in learning to cultivate, harness, and direct your own Qi for self-healing and sustained health. External Qigong will enable accomplished practitioners to project their energies into patients without touching them, often effecting miraculous healings.

UNDERSTANDING QI AND HEALTH

What Is the "Qi" in Qigong?

Qi is everything and everywhere: the primordial energy that creates life. In its pure form it is universal, undifferentiated energy. The concept of Qi is the underlying principle of Asian society as evidenced in feng shui, martial arts, and Oriental medicine. Qi is revered by the Chinese as the wellspring of life.

Humans are a natural conduit of Qi, which runs through invisible channels (meridians) in the body. Imagine an intricate electrical circuitry where energy courses throughout your physical being, carrying nourishment and providing pathways for communication between organs, the exterior and internal layers of the body, and the numerous networks within your system. Although Western scientists and doctors have tried to establish the correlations between acupuncture meridians and the circulatory, lymph, and nervous systems, there is no simple way to overlap these two very different approaches to viewing the human body. Western medicine concentrates on physiological function, while Chinese medicine focuses on energetics, incorporating physical, mental, emotional, and spiritual elements into the diagnostic and treatment process. Meridians are unique, intangible channels that serve as an important diagram of our energetic body. This intricate map of the human body has been utilized for thousands of years.

Chinese medical theory is based on the premise that disease occurs when there's an obstruction or imbalance of energy along these channels. Causes of illness can be attributed to a number of external factors such as trauma, exposure to the elements, or from internal disturbances related to stress or excessive emotions. Or it may simply be the wear and tear brought on by aging. The Chinese view the body as a hologram where all aspects affect the entire system (including the emotions) and cannot be separated out as in allopathic medicine. The organs are viewed as functional and energetic systems, intricately related with other parts of the body. Reference to an organ (both in Chinese medicine and in this book) encompasses its energetic function, association with other systems (i.e., each yin organ is paired with a yang organ), and the emotional and spiritual components. It does not refer solely to the defined physiological function as in Western medicine.

For example, if a woman comes to my clinic complaining of PMS, depression, and sore breasts, in Chinese medicine and Qigong healing, all of these symptoms can be related to stagnant Qi of the liver meridian. The liver itself is still healthy, but the energetic equilibrium has been disrupted. These imbalances can be regulated by inserting needles into the acupuncture points along the meridians or by practicing Qigong to regulate the energy flow. One of the most effective Qigong exercises, Push the Mountain, is a potent remedy for releasing anger and depression as well as harmonizing emotions for women suffering from PMS. (See chapter 13, PMS, p. 93 for a full explanation.)

The Yin/Yang Theory of Disease

Through observation and reflection, the Chinese witnessed the polarities inherent in the Universe and formulated the yin/yang concept. Everything is part of the whole, and although aspects may appear to be opposite, they are not polarized (as in our Western thinking)—rather, they represent a continuum. Night cannot exist without day, light without dark, nor soft without hard. Yin represents inward, cold, dark, hidden, feminine, and contracting qualities; yang is outward, hot, light, expansive, and masculine. Their relationship is symbolized in the Taoist tai chi symbol of yin/yang: yin and yang continually transform into one another without end, where the possibility of yin (as seen in the dark seed within the white) is poised within yang, and yang within yin.

In healing, we seek to balance these energies within the body. For example, during menopause a woman's yin fluids often become deficient, resulting in the manifestation of heat (yang) symptoms such as night sweats and hot flashes. To balance this, she will seek to build her yin and restore her natural yin/yang equilibrium.

To the Chinese, the human body is a microcosm of the Universe. They do not isolate symptoms nor seek to combat the causative pathogens. Rather, they look at the relationships within and around a person to understand the disharmony. A diagnosis is woven into a pattern by exploring the patient's complaints, medical history, emotions, relationships, environment, stressors, support system, constitution, and lifestyle. Only through this exploration can every aspect of the whole person be integrated into the creation of a treatment plan.

The causes of illness also vary. In ancient China the doctors believed that emotions played a significant role in wellness. The Seven Primary Emotions of sadness, grief, fear, fright, anger, elation, and worry were seen to adversely affect different organs. (This is discussed in more detail in chapter 8, Six Healing Sounds, and in chapter 7, Five-Element Healing). Environmental influences, such as wind, cold, damp, and dryness, may also infringe on a person's well-being, if she is unable to adapt or has a weak constitution. Many people, particularly the elderly, who have difficulty living in colder climates, cope by migrating to Florida or Arizona during the winter months. It's important to understand your own individual needs and adjust accordingly. Another important key to maintaining a healthy lifestyle is to avoid overindulgence in work, sex, alcohol, and food, as these excesses may cause disease. The main principle within Chinese medicine and Qigong is to seek moderation and balance in everything that you do.

THE THREE TREASURES

In the Oriental view, the way to vital health and immortality is to cultivate the "Three Treasures" known as the pillars of human life: *Qi, Jing,* and *Shen*. While *Qi* refers to life force, movement, and function in Chinese medicine, *Jing* is the life essence that includes our body fluids and primordial energies, and *Shen* is our spirit. All of these vital elements are nourished by Qigong practice.

Qi: Energy

Qi is our internal energy that propels the functions of the body. It is responsible for the metabolism, movement, and transformation of food into blood and other substances. It nourishes the organs, protects the body from external influences, and maintains overall performance. There are many different types of Qi, but the primary source of this energy is derived from the air that we breathe, the food we consume, and the spirit of our ancestors. We are born with a predetermined amount of Qi (congenital or

prenatal Qi), which is stored in the kidneys and holds our genetics and ancestral energy. As we mature, the amount of Qi available to us naturally diminishes; therefore incorporating Qigong into your day is like putting money into a retirement fund, a resource that will sustain you throughout your life.

Qi circulates in a rhythm similar to the circadian cycle, passing through each organ system at specific two-hour intervals. In medical Qigong practice, we use these designated times to diagnose the disharmony, as well as to optimize the healing effects. For example, often people will wake up coughing between 3:00 and 5:00 A.M. (the hours of the lung), or regularly get tired in the late afternoon during the kidney hours. Thus, if someone has a kidney imbalance, it is best to do the exercises during the kidney hours of 5:00 to 7:00 P.M. (see chapter 7, Five-Element Healing, p. 47). Unfortunately, this is usually not possible given the work ethic of the Western culture, but it is an ancient concept still utilized in Oriental medicine.

Jing: *Essence*

Jing holds the potential of our life: the deep juiciness of our sexuality and the underlying matrix of our development from the moment of our conception to our death. It forms the foundation of growth and reproduction, supplying essential body and reproductive fluids such as vaginal secretions, menstrual blood, and saliva, as well as the more subtle energies of our primal origins. This substance is stored in the kidneys and supports the seven-year development cycles of women. We are born with a certain amount of *Jing*, which accumulates through adolescence, peaks in our early twenties, and begins to deteriorate as we age. Thus, many age-related symptoms are associated with declining *Jing,* such as graying hair, osteoporosis, and poor memory.

Congenital (prenatal) *Jing* essence is formed from sexual union and is the substance that nourishes the embryo. Inherited from our parents, prenatal *Jing* carries the blueprint of our life and determines our basic constitution. The other source, postnatal *Jing,* is derived primarily from nutrition, but can be augmented by Qigong and Taoist sexual practices. *Jing* is very important to women and may be regarded as the "mother essence," possessed by women even if they don't give birth to a child. It enfolds our deep primal potential of birth. This nourishing essence needs to be honored like an opalescent pearl, for it is our precious gift. Restoring depleted *Jing* is harder than cultivating Qi, yet it is extremely important since this treasure controls bone growth, brain function, fertility, the reproductive cycle, and our mental-spiritual health.

Shen: *Spirit*

The emperor asked: "What is meant by the Shen, *the spirit?"*

Ch'i Po answered: "Let me discuss Shen, *the spirit."*

"What is the spirit? The spirit cannot be heard with the ear. The eye must be brilliant of perception and the heart must be open and attentive, and then the spirit is suddenly revealed through one's own consciousness. It cannot be expressed through the mouth; only the heart can express all that can be looked upon."[1]

Shen refers to our consciousness, mental faculties, and spiritual connection to life. It is our capacity for inner awareness and introspection. *Shen* encompasses the intuitive senses, as well as the "wise-woman self" that comprehends the entire Universe in her deepest unspoken being. *Shen* resides in the heart, but is witnessed through the sparkle in a person's eyes. Yet, despite the power and resilience of this energy, it can easily be disrupted by excessive emotions and result in anxiety, confusion, and mental disorders. Maintaining a positive attitude is therefore very important in Qigong healing, for when *Shen* is abundant, you will lead a strong, happy, and spiritually imbued life.

The Power of Blood

Although blood isn't one of the Three Treasures, it is an intricate part of a woman's life and consciousness. In Chinese medicine, blood is the substance (yin) aspect of Qi, nourishing and moistening the body. Liver blood, for example, moistens the eyes and keeps the tendons flexible. Blood also nourishes the heart and spirit so the mind can be calm. When the blood flow to the heart is deficient, it can induce insomnia, resulting in a restless mind.

While the heart is usually considered the main organ responsible for healthy blood circulation, there are many meridian systems involved in the supply and flow of blood. Blood originates from the transformation of nutrients in the stomach and spleen, which are then circulated throughout the body by the heart. The liver stores blood at rest and the spleen holds the blood in the vessels. All three of these yin meridians—heart, liver, and spleen—are extremely important to a woman's menstrual health and illustrate the mutual interdependence of all the organs and body systems.

QIGONG PRACTITIONERS, particularly the Taoists, aspire to cultivate the Three Treasures to attain a peaceful mind, immortality, and spiritual awareness. The Taoist tenet is that "*Qi* is like the root and *Jing* is like the trunk of the tree. If the root is not deep, it can easily be pulled, and if the trunk is not strong, then it will fall. When one is able to firmly store *Qi* and guard *Jing*, one will be able to attain longevity."[2] By cultivating and storing Qi (our life energy), nourishing *Jing* (our sexual and primal juiciness), and refining *Shen* (our spiritual essence), we promote a synergistic approach to truly harmonize the body, mind, and spirit.

3

Exploring Qi

Perhaps the only limits to the human mind
are those we believe in.

—Willis Harman

Before the advent of quantum physics, the Chinese had formulated that all things are composed of energy particles that are constantly spiraling in space, connecting and influencing each other throughout the Universe. This dynamic life force energy, called Qi, is what you will learn to cultivate and utilize in Qigong.

ENERGETIC BOUNDARIES

Energetic healing is a vast subject, yet there are some basic principles to be aware of as you embark on this path of self-healing. We often unconsciously connect to others through energetic threads that extend outward from our body like a web, attaching to those we love and our families. This concept is particularly rel-

evant for women, since they are more likely to overextend themselves for the welfare of others. If you are unaware of your energetic boundaries, this behavior can result in fatigue and illness.

To discover where you are losing energy, simply ask yourself: Are you ever tired or do you feel drained after being with someone? Do others invade your space at work, and you are reluctant to say anything? Do you have a friend or relative who regularly confides in you, going into great detail about their life drama of the week? As natural caretakers and "mothers," women often have difficulty establishing boundaries or saying no. It is our essential nature to give, yet we may find ourselves feeling exhausted or resentful. Learning to become more responsive to these energy fields will help you reclaim your Qi.

The first step is to become aware of your actions and notice when or how you lose momentum during the day. This will make it easier to attend to your energetic boundaries so you may bolster your Qi when necessary. As you do Qigong, you will harness life force energy and store this Qi in your *dantian*. The stances are particularly powerful in strengthening your energy field both internally and externally, especially if you create the intention to magnify your energy body. As the Chinese say, "Where you set your mind, the Qi will follow."

Qi Awareness Exercise

Though most people can't see it, you can easily experience the presence of Qi. Through a variety of simple exercises, you will become familiar with your energetic body that vibrates within and around you. This subtle field carries the blueprint of your physical health; disharmonies show up here first, before they impact your physical body. Qigong activates and heals this force field, reestablishing harmony to stave off disease.

Begin by trying to sense the energy field surrounding your being; palpate the space about one to three inches away from your body with your palms. It's very subtle. Close your eyes to help you focus inward. Experiment with sensations at different distances from your body (described more fully in the Qi Ball exercise that follows). Where is your field the strongest? Where does it end? Does it seem to have a boundary? Visualize a vibrant field (or aura) a few inches from your body, pulsating with light. Slowly expand it out a few feet and then farther out to fill the room. Then gradually bring your energy back close to your body and remain quiet for a few minutes. What do you notice? Do you feel different?

Now walk around the room and imagine an egg of energy wrapped around your body, enfolding you in its healing light. Does this feel comforting, safe, relaxing? How does your energy change when you get near others? Do you sense it streaming out or wanting to merge with another's Qi?

Try walking around with your field wide open, expanded to encompass everyone in the room, and then retract your energy back into your body. Notice your internal responses. Come back to your original position and close your eyes again. How did your energy change? Were there any shifts in your awareness and which felt more comfortable? How do you usually go out into the world? Wide open? Contracted? Are you even aware of your energy boundaries?

Explore this in your daily life to discover how you use your Qi and where it dissipates. This is especially important if you have a chronic illness or struggle with fatigue. Improved health could be as simple as discerning where your energy lines are connected and consciously pulling them back to nourish yourself.

Exploring the Qi Ball

Stand or sit in a relaxed manner, take a few deep belly breaths and exhale fully through your mouth. You may want to exhale with a loud sigh or make sounds to relieve tension. Now rub your palms together vigorously until they're warm. Gradually move your palms apart until they are about six inches away from one another.

Close your eyes and attune to any sensations between your palms. If you don't feel anything, gradually bring your palms closer together until you can sense a springiness in the air between your hands. Take a few moments to explore your "ball" of energy. Keep your shoulders relaxed and breathe. Once you've connected with some impression, move your hands in and out slowly as though you are playing an accordion. Does the feeling change? Is there a difference when your palms are two inches or a foot apart? When you are finished, slowly open your hands out to the side and observe where the sensations subside.

I usually begin my classes with this exercise and most people discover a magnetic pulse, as if there's a pressure between their palms. Others feel tingling or heat—one eight-year-old exclaimed, "It's like cotton candy!" This is a fun exercise to share with your family and everyone will have a different experience, often changing each time you do it. Some days your field will be expansive and large while other times it might be indiscernible. One thing that's constant in life is change!

Exploring Qi with a Partner

Sit facing your partner and raise your palms so they are mirroring your partner's palms; leave about a foot of space between your hands. Decide who will be the Sender and who will be the Receiver. The Sender begins by experimenting with different ways to emit Qi through their palms to their partner. Imagine drawing energy up from the Earth (yin essence) and send it out through your hands, or filter it down from the Universe (yang essence) through the top of your head. Or you can simply concentrate on sending the energy out your hands to the other person. Close your eyes and remember to breathe as you experience this exchange. Switch roles, repeat the process, and share your experience with your partner.

Another fun experiment involves transmitting a color. I suggest that you stick to simple colors like red, yellow, blue, green, purple, or orange to make it easier on your partner. Often in a group, there's a joker who will send mauve or change colors midstream. I once had a man send his partner a rainbow!

Along with being fun, these explorations also help to attune you to the energy you will utilize for self-healing in this book. Qi is the basic element of Qigong, so it's helpful to become aware of the sensations as you begin. If you find yourself getting tense or concentrating too hard to learn a movement, then return to the Qi Ball exercise to reacquaint yourself with the feel of the energy.

Remember: the overall intention of Qigong is to become more energetic while remaining relaxed. This practice is not about perfecting the details and performing precise movements as you would with tai chi or other disciplines (such as yoga). It's more important to move with the energy and follow your body's innate wisdom. Dr. Wu and I enjoy doing free-form Qigong by the ocean, tuning into the rhythms around us. No form, no boundaries, just pure essence in movement or stillness.

4

Activating Your Energy

QIGONG BREATHING AND
WARM-UP EXERCISES

There is a way of breathing that's a shame and a suffocation.
And there's another way of expiring, a love breath
that lets you open infinitely.

—RUMI

IT IS AN ANCIENT Chinese belief that we are created from the union of Heavenly and Earthly Qi; thus it is important to honor and cultivate these energies through focused breathing. When we are born, we are spanked into consciousness to grasp our first taste of air; yet from that point on most of us remain unaware of our respiration, breathing in a shallow and irregular manner. Qigong reminds us of our dependence on breathing and its inherent potential, for it is respiration that changed our whole physiology at birth and keeps us alive today.

QIGONG BREATHING

Qigong breathing is most commonly focused in the energy center of the body called the *dantian* (*dan* means "elixir" and *tian* translates to "field"). The Taoists believe that the *dantian* is the alchemical cauldron where we gather energies to create the elixir of long life and health (symbolized by actual cauldrons found in Chinese Taoist temples). The lower *dantian* is located a couple of inches below the umbilicus on the abdomen. Focused breathing, drawn into and exhaled from this center, is the key to medical Qigong and will be the *dantian* that I primarily refer to throughout this book.

Since this is the natural center of gravity in the body, many Qigong movements originate from this focal point. As you perform the exercises, you will harness and store nourishing Qi in this area. With practice you will learn to direct the Qi to different parts of your body for healing or to tap into this energy storehouse to attain vitality, increased sexuality, and an overall sense of well-being.

There are three *dantians* in the body. The lower *dantian* (described earlier) is the power center most commonly utilized in Qigong practice and serves as the body's reservoir of energy. The middle *dantian* sits between the breasts in the middle of the chest. This is important for lung and heart function as well as distributing Qi throughout the body. Respiration for the breast Qigong in this book activates the middle *dantian*. Some meditative Qigong forms also focus on the middle *dantian* (since it's close to the heart) to expand one's compassion and love. The upper *dantian* corresponds with the third eye point located between the eyebrows on the forehead. This is where the *Shen* (or spiritual consciousness) is concentrated and is used to develop heightened awareness. (See fig. 4.1.)

In addition to the three *dantians*, women also

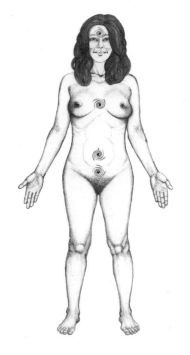

[4.1]

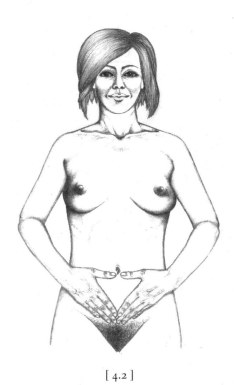

[4.2]

have an energy center called the Uterine Palace. (Even if your uterus has been removed, the energetics of this area are still intact.) The Uterine Palace is found by placing your palms on your lower abdomen, with your thumbs on your belly button and your index fingers forming the apex of a triangle with your fingers pointing down toward your pubis. The point underneath your index fingers is the Uterine Palace, while the ovaries are under the middle fingers (with fingers spread apart). (See fig. 4.2.)

Women may resonate more with this feminine energy center, since as women we are procreators with life emerging from our wombs. Whether we have children or not, the potential of birth lies within us, and thus the Uterine Palace is the source for healing and revitalizing the reproductive organs. Since the Uterine Palace is a valuable component in women's Qigong healing, I've included exercises to activate this important energy center throughout the book.

Basic Qigong (Dantian) Breathing

Stand with your feet shoulder-width apart, knees relaxed (this can also be done while seated or lying down). Place a few fingers on the lower *dantian*, about a couple of inches below the belly button and press gently to bring your awareness to this area. All of the breathing is done through the nose. As you breathe in, gently expand your stomach outward as if blowing up a balloon. Imagine taking the Qi in through your nostrils and visualize it moving down to energize your *dantian* with each inhalation. On the exhalation, contract the belly and allow the air to move out naturally. Your breath should be deep, slow, gentle, and rhythmic, like ocean waves.

This is the basic Qigong breathing (also called *dantian* breathing) that will be referred to throughout this book. Begin by practicing this technique for one to three minutes in the morning and evening, and as you become comfortable with it, add the following refinements:

1. Place the tip of your tongue on the roof of your mouth, softly touch the upper palate right behind the teeth. This connects the conception and governing meridians, which circulate in an orbit along the midline of the body (front and back). Instead of running up the spine like in yoga, the energy in Qigong is circular, nourishing the body and mind.

2. Next, gently pull up on the anus with each exhalation. This prevents the energy from leaking out.

These two adjustments are done in most of the Qigong exercises, so it is helpful to acquaint yourself with this basic breathing until it feels natural and becomes automatic. You may feel dizzy, light-headed, or nauseous when you first begin because you may not be used to taking in so much oxygen. Just continue the practice and these symptoms will subside.

QIGONG WARM-UPS

After you've spent a few moments concentrating on *dantian* breathing to quiet the mind and body, proceed with a few warm-up exercises to activate your Qi before doing a full Qigong routine.

Whole-Body Pat

This stimulates the entire body for increased energy and circulation and is great to do in the early morning or anytime you need to recharge.

1. Comfortably extend one arm out with palm facing upward. Using your other hand, pat down the length of the arm (beginning at the shoulder) to the hand, and then rotate the palm of the extended arm so it is facing downward, and continue up the outer arm from the hand to the shoulder. Repeat the process on the opposite arm.

2. Using the same patting motion, move both hands simultaneously from the chest (including the armpit), along the torso (stimulating the digestive organs), down to the outer thighs and legs to the feet. Then come up the inner legs, patting around the knees and up the thighs.

3. Stimulate the buttocks by softly pounding with loose fists and then pat up the back on either side of the spine.

4. Curl your hands into claws and tap the back of the neck; continue the same action up to the vertex of your head and around your scalp.

5. Gently tap your fingers on your face, especially around the eyes and sinuses.

6. End by shaking out your hands and whole body.

Hip Rotation

Rotating the hips keeps the Qi and blood flowing in the pelvis and loosens the lower back. This is good to do throughout the day, particularly if you sit at a desk.

1. Put your thumbs on both hips (facing front) and place four fingers on your kidney area (on the back, around your waist).

2. Slowly rotate your hips in circles, breathing in as you move forward and exhaling as you circle back.

3. Keep your torso relatively upright without leaning over as you circle.

Circle nine times in each direction.

Shoulder Shrugging

This invigorating exercise awakens the Qi in the whole body, increases internal energy and trims the waist. Perform this in the morning to really get yourself going! My teacher was challenged by his students to continue this exercise for ten minutes, since it's difficult to sustain for even a few minutes. Delighted by the dare, he did Shoulder Shrugging for ten minutes a day for two weeks and lost two inches off his waist!

1. Stand with your feet about shoulder-width apart. Be sure to wear sneakers to support your feet while doing this exercise.

2. Raise up on your toes and alternately drop one heel down, then pop back up as the other heel comes down. There should be a spring action to this movement with the emphasis on elongating the body upward as you drop down.

3. When you feel comfortable with the foot-spring action, then alternately rotate your shoulders up and back in circles. (See fig. 4.3.)

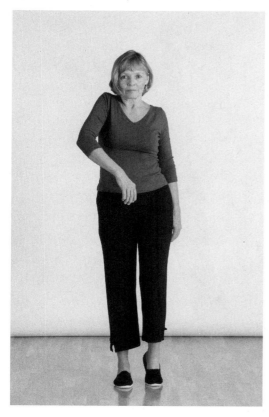

[4.3]

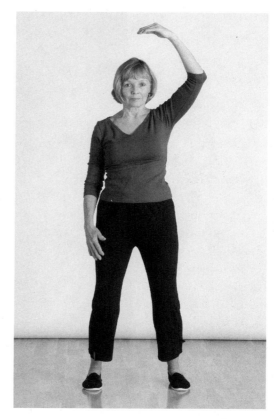

[4.4]

This exercise is very energizing. Begin with one minute and work up to three minutes.

Simple Snake Movements

The Simple Snake Movements activate and move the Qi throughout your body, and strengthen your shoulders and arms. Perform each of the following snake movements eight to twenty-four times a day, depending on your fitness level.

OVERHEAD CIRCLE

This movement loosens tension in the shoulder and upper back and elongates the side of the torso.

1. Alternately circle your arms overhead, front to back.
2. Keep your arms rounded in a crescent moon shape as you stretch them above your head.

Continue this snake stretch for one minute or eight to twenty-four times. (See fig. 4.4.)

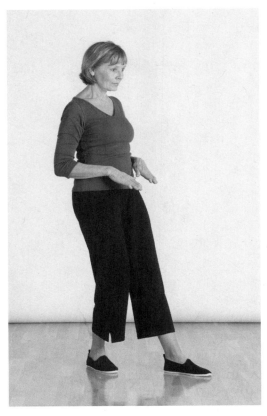

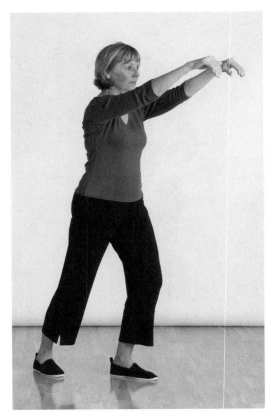

[4.5]

[4.6]

BIG QI BALL

1. Turn about 45 degrees to your side and imagine there's a large beach ball in front of your chest. Circle your hands around the perimeter of this imaginary sphere with your palms about a foot apart, facing downward.

Inhale

2. Draw your hands upward along your torso from your lower abdomen to your chest. Palms face your body. (See fig. 4.5.)

Exhale

3. Then extend your arms outward in front of your chest, drawing a semicircle from your chest to your lower abdomen. Imagine tracing a ball in front of your torso throughout this exercise. Allow your body to move with this motion, rocking back and forth as you circle your arms in front of you. (See fig. 4.6.) Now turn 45 degrees to the other side and repeat.

The rhythm of this movement should be relaxing and entrancing.

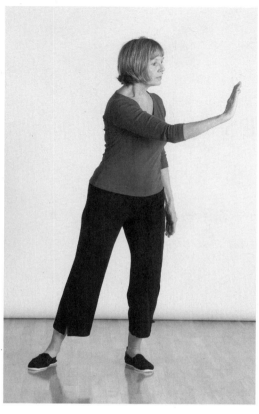

[4.7]

SIDE PUSH

1. Facing center, bring your right hand in front of you with your palm parallel to your body, fingers together, pointing toward the sky.

2. Press your hand from right to left, keeping it at chest level as you twist slightly at the waist. (See fig. 4.7.)

3. As you reach the left side, let your right hand drop back to your right side while the left hand raises and presses in front from left to right.

4. The arms alternate, tracing a half circle out in front of you as you turn from side to side.

Gathering Your Qi

1. After you've awakened your Qi, stand in Basic Qigong Stance (chapter 5, Stances, p. 28) with your palms over your *dantian*. Rest your right palm a couple of inches below your belly button and lay your left one on top.

2. Close your eyes and focus your attention on your energy center.

3. Take at least ten deep abdominal breaths to calm your mind and set your intentions for your healing.

Remember: Qigong is about balancing body, mind, and spirit, so this preliminary pose attunes you inward to quiet your thoughts and connect with your Qi.

5
Stances

He who overcomes others has force;
he who overcomes himself is strong.

—Lao-tzu

QIGONG STANCES harness internal energy for the development of stamina and a resilient immune system. They are a key element in all schools of Qigong and build strength and focused attention. A comprehensive Qigong program, whether to maintain health or cure illness, should include at least one stance, along with gentle movements and meditation.

QIGONG STANCES

Basic Qigong Stance

This is the standing position that will be referred to in most of the exercises described in this book, unless otherwise noted.

1. Begin by standing with your feet parallel, about shoulder-width apart, toes pointing forward.

2. Bend your knees slightly but make sure your knees don't extend beyond your toes, which could cause knee discomfort.

3. Relax your shoulders and let your arms hang by your sides. If you view yourself in a mirror, your back should be relatively straight, except for the natural curve in your lower back. Slightly tuck your chin so the top of your head (acupuncture point Governing Vessel 20) is open to the heavens. Imagine a string pulling you upward. At the same time, visualize roots anchoring you down into the ground through your feet.

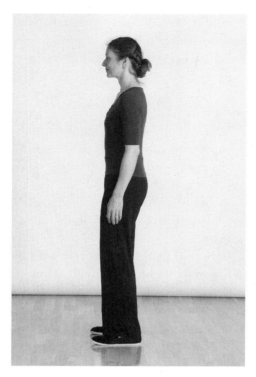

[5.1]

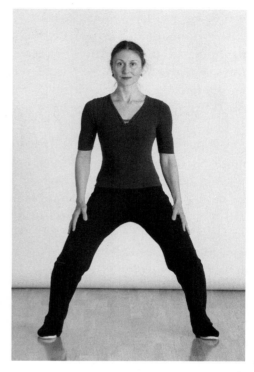

[5.2]

4. Remain relaxed, open, and expansive. It might take a while to become accustomed to this stance, but as you practice it will feel more natural. (See fig. 5.1.)

Stand in this position as you practice your Qigong *dantian* breathing at the beginning of each session. This posture is also used between exercises to direct energy back into your *dantian*.

Horse Stance

This is a martial arts stance that is used for more rigorous Qigong exercises.

1. Stand with your feet approximately 3 feet apart with your toes pointing forward or slightly out.

2. Squat down as if riding a horse, with your knees bent comfortably, not extending over your toes. Remember to keep your back relatively straight and make sure your buttocks do not protrude out behind you.

3. Imagine you have roots extending from your feet, grounding your energy into the Earth. In this posture, I picture my body as a willow tree with roots tethered in the soil and my upper torso flexible and yielding like the willow swaying in the wind. (See fig. 5.2.)

This is a power stance. You should feel strong in your legs so no one could topple you over. To test if you're balanced and rooted, have someone try to push you over with moderate force. If you're unfocused or if your energy is still in your upper body, you will be displaced or fall over. This is a fun exercise to do with kids and teaches them the power of intention and focus.

Initially you may lack the stamina to hold the Horse Stance, so you could begin with an easier variation: the Modified Horse Stance involves holding your legs slightly closer together in a modified squat.

Hugging the Tree Pose and Three-Circles Stance

A common position is the Hugging the Tree Pose. This is the foundational stance in most Qigong schools to build internal strength, and I've seen people of all ages doing variations of this posture in parks here and in China.

The Three-Circles Stance is the posture I had to hold for thirty minutes before Dr. Wu would take me on as an apprentice. In the beginning my legs shook and my arms got heavy and tired, while sweat dripped down my face. During the first two weeks of practice I got dizzy and sometimes nauseous, but eventually the symptoms disappeared. It took me about four months of dedicated practice to hold this position for thirty minutes. It was tedious and difficult, but in the end I had thighs of steel!

Hugging the Tree Pose

1. Stand in the Basic Qigong Stance with your knees bent comfortably. If you're in good shape, you can bend deeper into the stance and spread your feet a bit wider.

2. Raise your arms up in front as if holding a big Qi ball (like a beach ball) at the level of your heart.

3. Face your palms toward you, with about a foot of space between your hands. Your elbows are slightly pointing down to the ground and your shoulders are relaxed.

4. Tuck your chin slightly and imagine you have a cord attached at the apex of your head tugging your spine upward.

5. At the same time visualize this cord extending from the bottom of your spine down into the Earth, rooting you to the ground. Feel the subtle spinal stretch going both downward and upward simultaneously.

6. Remain standing as you do deep *dantian* breathing.

Keep your mind quiet and concentrate on inhaling into the *dantian;* allow the energies to spread throughout your body on the exhalation. Relax so your Qi can flow smoothly. If you notice places of discomfort, this is where your Qi is blocked. Envision healing energies soothing these areas as you exhale the pain from your body, then return to your *dantian* breathing to harmonize your entire being.

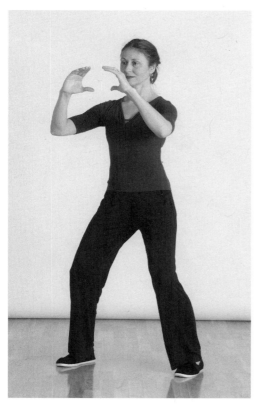

[5.3]

The Three-Circles Stance

This is a more powerful and difficult stance for activating your energy. The three circles are created by your thighs, arms, and hands.

I. Stand in Horse Stance with your knees bent at a 135-degree angle. Although this is the ultimate goal, if you have leg or knee problems or you are weak in general, then only bend slightly (in a Modified Horse Stance) until you're comfortable.

2. Circle your arms in front of your body in the same way described in the Hugging the Tree Pose. However, instead of having your palms facing your body, create another circle with your hands, as if you were holding a small ball, about level with your nose. (See fig. 5.3.)

3. Peer through this second circle with an unfocused gaze or close your eyes as you concentrate on *dantian* breathing.

Slowly build up your stamina. Begin with standing one minute, then three, and gradually increase the duration in small, incremental steps up to ten minutes or longer, depending on your fitness goals.

Awkward Stance

This is a more advanced pose, which stimulates the three yin leg meridians—the kidney, spleen, and liver—increasing Qi flow up the inner legs into the pelvis. This stance is used to restore depleted immune systems, to cure gynecological/urinary diseases, and to augment balance.

I. Stand with your heels touching and your toes splayed outward, forming a right angle with your feet.
Inhale
2. Lift up on your toes, while keeping your heels together.
3. Simultaneously raise your arms upward to the sides, then circle them to the front of your body, and end by holding them in prayer position in front of your heart. (If you're averse to holding your hands in the prayer position, then create a circle with your arms in front, palms

face down, and middle fingers touching in front of your chest).

Exhale

4. While remaining on your toes, sink into bent knees, with your back straight (and an imaginary string pulling your head into the clouds), as you concentrate on deep *dantian* breathing. (See fig. 5.4.)

Begin by standing for one minute, then for three minutes, and slowly build up your endurance until you can stand comfortably for ten minutes, which is quite difficult.

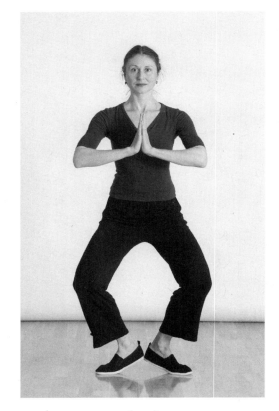

[5.4]

6

Meditations and Visualizations

A man does not seek to see himself in running water,
but in still water. For only what is itself still
can impart stillness to others.

—CHUANG-TSE

MEDITATION IS AN integral component of Qigong, training the mind to concentrate and focus. By slowing down the incessant chatter of the mind, you will learn to direct your attention to deeply connect with the present moment. This requires practice and patience to drop your worries, plans, and thoughts—and just sit, without any agenda. Using a myriad of methods such as breathing, counting, walking, or mantras, the mind will become calm and settled. You don't have to embrace a particular religion to incorporate meditation into your daily life—it is simply a matter of becoming mindful of your actions, thoughts, and behav-iors to generate more compassion and kindness for yourself and others.

The Tibetan master Tulku Thondup wrote, "If we cluttered up our homes with too much furniture we would have no place to live. If our minds are cluttered with plans, concerns, thoughts, and emotional patterns, then we have no space for our true selves."[1] Personally, I feel meditation is my time away from worldly distractions where I can be alone and commune with the Divine. I relish these moments of silence, bathed in serenity. The process can take on many forms, but the intention is still to touch one's essential nature. Once you embody this awareness, you can draw upon a profound inner peace to guide you.

MEDITATION BASICS

Many people have the image of a yogi or monk sitting in a cave in an austere posture of devout meditation, but there are many ways to adapt this practice to your life. Some people have difficulty sitting still, so choose one of the following meditations that fit with your character and lifestyle.

First designate an area in your home that's quiet, without distractions. Create your own unique space, employing uplifting symbols, such as pictures of teachers, spiritual masters, and loved ones, along with inspirational objects. Design an altar where you will want to come to find peace and solace. This can be as simple as a small table in the corner of your bedroom adorned with a candle or flower, or a more elaborate shrine. Whatever you decide, be sure that it enriches your soul.

Before you begin meditating, turn off the TV, phone, and music, so you can sit in silence. This is essential, since most people today are bombarded with technology all day long and have forgotten the stillness of silence. Meditation (and silence) will help calm your nervous system and relax your entire body and mind. You may want to commence your meditations by lighting a candle or sounding a chime or singing bowl. Be imaginative and enjoy your personal ritual.

Sit on a meditation pillow (called a *zafu*), meditation bench, or in a straight-backed chair where your feet can comfortably reach the floor.

Try to sit with a straight back to allow the Qi to flow easily, without restraint. Rest your hands on your lap, with the back of your right hand cradled in your left palm, with thumbs lightly touching to form a circle. Be relaxed but not slumped, soften your belly, relax your jaw, and release facial tension.

Begin with a few deep breaths: inhale through your nose and exhale tension out your mouth; add a few sighs to discharge any constrained Qi. Then allow your breath to become soft and quiet, without controlling the flow. Either close your eyes or keep them half-open with a soft gaze, focusing a few feet in front of you. I find I prefer to close my eyes to relax them after a day of computer glare, yet I keep more awake with them open. Do whatever feels most comfortable for you.

Mindfulness Meditation

"Breathing in, I calm my body.
Breathing out, I smile.
Dwelling in the present moment
I know this is a wonderful moment."[2]
— THICH NHAT HANH

Begin by simply watching your breath. Follow the rise and fall of your chest or belly, or notice the sensation of the air moving in and out, brushing against your nostrils as you breathe. Silently repeat the words "breathing in— breathing out" to help keep yourself focused. Your mind will wander; simply bring it back and once again notice your breath. As one of my meditation teachers instructed, a beginning practice is like training a puppy to pee on paper. Just keep leading the puppy (your mind) back to the paper (your breath); remember to refocus on your breath each time your mind wanders off, over and over again. Start by sitting for ten minutes and gradually work up to twenty to forty minutes. Remember: a short, concentrated meditation is better than an hour of monkey mind.

TRANQUIL QIGONG MEDITATIONS

The following meditations and visualizations are designed to address certain conditions and different personality types. Explore any or all of these meditations and adopt the one that suits you. In the women's self-healing chapters (part 3), there will be specific recommended meditations based on medical Qigong principles to create an optimal healing plan for each imbalance.

Five-Eight Meditation

The Five-Eight Meditation reduces stress and is a simple exercise for those who have difficulty with meditation. I've prescribed this breathing technique with beneficial results to patients with hypertension, cancer, digestive problems, and chronic illness. You can do this breathing anytime during the day or in the midst of a stressful situation. I find it instantly relaxing when I'm on a plane, driving on city freeways, or preparing for public speaking.

Take a few deep breaths and expel any tension out your mouth. Sighing helps relieve pent-up stress. Then begin the meditation by gently inhaling through the nose and slowly counting to five. Exhale (through the nose) to the count of eight. The prolonged exhalation relaxes the sympathetic fight-or-flight response, calming the nervous system into a deeper level of relaxation. Continue with this restful breathing to a count of five-in (inhalation) and eight-out (exhalation); concentrate on the rhythm of your breath, allowing all other thoughts to float by, without attending to them. Sit for ten to twenty minutes.

Sea Meditation

This is a regulating meditation to help you calm down and let go of worries. It's especially recommended for artistic personalities and those who tend to be emotionally sensitive.

Assume a meditation posture and take a few deep, soothing breaths. Close your eyes and imagine the sea's rolling swell. Hear the soothing rhythm of the ocean in your imagination. If you live by the sea, sit and listen to the waves, allowing the continuous drone to become your mantra.

You may also begin this meditation by reflecting on the qualities of the ocean. One Chinese tale recounts that Kuan Yin, the goddess of compassion, listened to the sea and attained enlightenment. When contemplating the tumultuous nature of the ocean in relation to life's challenges, she realized that a deep inner calm always exists underneath turbulence, just as with the sea. The mind is no different: there is an unwavering essence of our true self that is untouched by the waves of life. Dive beneath the surface of your life, and relax into the profound inner peace amidst the distractions of daily activity.

Dunhuang *Meditation*

This meditation was reputedly gathered from the famous Magao grottoes in Dunhuang, China, which contain some of the most impressive examples of Chinese Buddhist cave art and sculptures. First inspired by the vision of a monk in 366 C.E., the sandstone cave temples were part of a rich cultural center along the Silk Road where Buddhist monks and craftsmen lived and worked for many centuries. The caves were adorned with paintings, including documentation of early healing exercises and meditations, which are now housed in museums around the world.

Dunhuang is a cleansing meditation; by expelling negativity, it clears the body of tension and calms the mind. This is particularly helpful when you're feeling overwhelmed or if you've been absorbing other people's energies and problems.

1. Sit on a firm chair with your legs crossed at the ankles or stand with one leg crossed over the other.
2. Slightly lift your arms away from your sides with your elbows angled outward about 6 inches from your body.
3. Create an incomplete circle with your thumb and index fingers (as if holding an egg) and spread and bend the other fingers like talons. (See fig. 6.1.)
4. The space between the thumb and index finger faces the ground to allow for the negative energies to flow out of your body and into the Earth. It's helpful to tense the fingers to create the talon effect, but then relax your hands while maintaining the position.

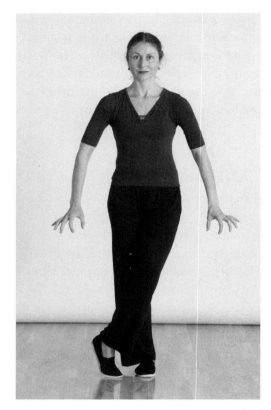

[6.1]

Sit or stand for five to ten minutes doing *dantian* breathing.

Ren Chong *Meditation for Women*

The *Ren Chong* Meditation nourishes the Qi and blood of a woman, and is especially beneficial for perimenopause, menopause, poor digestion, reproductive problems, or PMS. Perform this breathing practice after completing your Qigong routine.

There are two meridians that are particularly important to women since they govern the flow of blood and Qi in the body and dispel stagnation such as abdominal bloating, menstrual pain, or tumors. *Ren mai* controls Qi circulation in the front of the body and is called the "conception vessel" since it is vital to reproduction. It originates in the pelvis, emerges at the perineum, and goes up the centerline of the body to the chin, where an internal branch circles the mouth and ends under the eyes. *Ren mai* supports the yin and directly affects the entire menstrual cycle from menarche through menopause.

Chong mai originates in the kidneys, passes through the uterus, and follows the kidney meridian up the abdomen to below the breasts. It then ascends internally through the chest and throat to end at the mouth. It's considered a primordial meridian, one of the first to develop in utero. Called the "sea of blood," it influences deep blood circulation and regulates the uterus, menstruation, and nourishes the blood along with *ren mai*. Although it spreads Qi throughout the body, its primary influence is in the abdomen, uterus, chest, and heart.

1. Sit comfortably with hands resting on your thighs.

Inhale

2. Bring your breath down to your *dantian* —imagine the energy traveling from your nostrils down to your belly.

Exhale

3. Visualize the Qi sinking down to your perineum (the spot between your anus and vagina) and then rising up the center of your body to right below your eyes. This may feel awkward at first, but it will become easier as

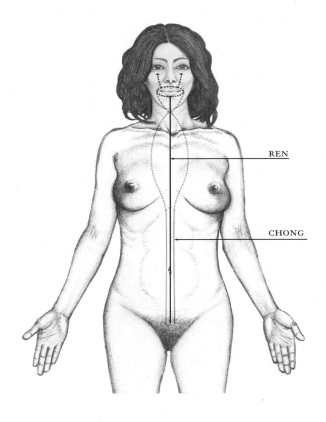

[6.2]

you practice. Keep the visualization simple by following the flow up the torso, through the throat, to the eyes. (The specific details of the meridians are more for your reference.) If you're directing the energy correctly, your hands will warm up from the increase in circulation. (See fig. 6.2.)

Continue for ten minutes. Then rub your palms together vigorously until they're warm and place them on any area that needs healing or comforting.

7

Five-Element Healing

Human beings follow the Earth,
the Earth follows heaven, heaven follows the Tao,
and the Tao follows Nature.

—LAO-TZU

ACQUAINTING YOURSELF with the essence of the Five Elements will deepen your experience of Qigong and heighten your connection with Nature within and around you. You will learn to recognize the different associations of the elements (such as emotions) in relation to your health and balance them through the practice of simple exercises for each element. These suggestions can be incorporated into your daily Qigong routine or done separately (like lying in the sun to gather yang Qi vitality described in the Fire Element section.)

UNDERSTANDING THE FIVE ELEMENTS/ORGAN SYSTEMS

Throughout this book I talk about different organ systems (which are part of the Five Element Theory); this overview will illustrate the relationship of many emotional and physical imbalances, and thus help focus your personal healing. Each element has a different signature and the following descriptions will give you an idea of how emotions can affect your body. As you become more attuned to energy through your Qigong practice, sense where you feel various emotions in your body. How are they affecting your well-being and expression in the world? This exploration, in combination with performing the Six Healing Sounds exercises, will help you develop an internal awareness for deeper self-healing and disease prevention (see chapter 8, Six Healing Sounds).

The ancient Chinese lived with the knowledge that humans are inseparable from Nature. They believed their survival depended on the environment, so they became attuned to the seasons and phases inherent in the natural world around them. Early Chinese healers realized that these cycles and natural qualities were also infused into human life and concluded that our bodies are composed of five elements: Wood, Fire, Earth, Metal, and Water. Through extensive observation, a whole healing system was developed, associating these elements with corresponding body organs, emotions, seasons, healing colors, foods, and other attributes. By aligning with these energies of Nature, it is possible to prevent and heal disease, as well as reconnect with our innate spiritual essence.

Using the Five Elements system in Chinese medicine for diagnosis and treatment is very complex. However, some of the basic tenets are easily adopted for general Qigong treatment. The Chinese translation of Five Elements denotes movement: "five things in action, moving in relationship to one another." In healing, the concept is that the organ systems are interconnected, each affecting the other in continuous transformation.

The Creation Cycle (also called mother-son cycle or *Shen* phase) illustrates the genesis of the elements. Water feeds the Wood element to become forests, which are cut for fuel to create Fire, and then the decomposing ashes form Earth, which compresses to create Metal, and then liquefies into the minerals supporting Water. It's an unending cycle where the mother feeds and nourishes her son (daughter): Water is the mother of Wood; Wood, in turn, is the mother of Fire; Fire is the mother of Earth; Earth is the mother of Metal; and finally Metal is the mother of Water. Every element is inseparable, one merging into the next in this continuing circle of cocreation. (See fig. 7.1.)

Another direction of energy flow is expressed as the Control Cycle, which keeps these elements in check (the star within the Creation Cycle Circle in fig. 7.1). Water controls Fire, Fire transforms Metal (by liquefying it), Metal cuts Wood; Wood holds the Earth in containment; and Earth shores up the Water (in dams). In acupuncture and Qigong therapy, these generating or inhibiting relationships are used during treatment. For example, when there's a weakness in an organ, we'll tonify (nourish) the mother organ to assist the ailing organ (the child). If you had heart problems, we would not only address the heart and its associated meridians, but we would also treat the liver to generate more supportive energy (mother-son cycle) and the kidneys to balance Qi for nurturing the heart (Control Cycle).

To broaden your understanding of these elements, I've designed a chart for quick reference at the beginning of each element description. Included in each section is the signature of the

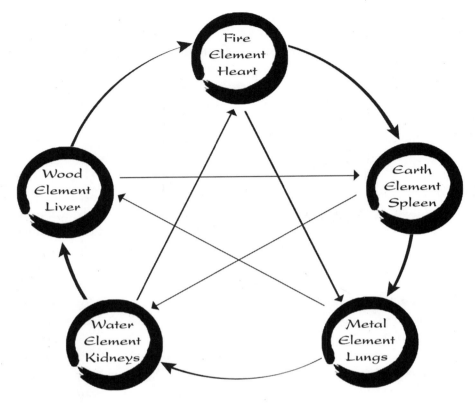

[7.1]

element as I experience it, the associated organs and emotions, and suggestions for healing the element with Qigong (or color visualization) and foods. You can use this awareness to attune to the appropriate element as you practice the Six Healing Sounds, or the suggested exercises can be added to any sequence. How do you decide which element would be beneficial? If you have an imbalance in either of the associated organs, or if you tend to experience one emotion more than the others, then add this element's exercise to your routine a couple of times a week.

WOOD ELEMENT

Organ Systems:	Liver and Gallbladder
Color:	Spring Green
Emotion:	Anger, Depression vs. Gentleness, Patience
Season:	Spring
Direction:	East
Hours:	Gallbladder 11 P.M.–1 A.M.; Liver 1–3 A.M.
Taste:	Sour
Sensory Organ:	Eyes (Sight)

The Nature of Wood

The tree symbolizes the Wood element with its roots reaching deep into the Earth and branches outstretched toward the sun. The trunk is strong and firm, yet bends with wind and weather. She is both yielding and strong, holding ancestral knowledge in her rings that record the ages. From a vulnerable, small seed within the Earth, a sapling can sometimes grow to a momentous size, like the redwoods—a symbol of growth, longevity, and ancient wisdom. Plants sustain our life by emitting oxygen and cleansing the atmosphere; they are an integral part of our survival, providing warmth, shelter, food, medicine, and beauty.

The liver and gallbladder are the organ systems corresponding to the Wood element. The gallbladder is primarily a digestive organ while the liver has a multitude of tasks. The liver meridian maintains the health of tendons and ligaments, which keep us resilient as they hold our skeletal structure together. Just as the limbs of a tree need proper nourishment to grow and extend, we need a healthy Wood element to be truly flexible in our physique. The sense organ nourished by Wood is the eyes, so the liver is almost always addressed in vision problems. This also encompasses our inner spiritual sight: like a tree, we want to remain graceful and yielding to life's challenges, rooted by our deepest knowing.

The liver also controls the smooth flow of Qi throughout the body, as well as the circulation and storage of blood, so this meridian is particularly important in women's gynecological health. Anger, depression, and frustration easily disrupt this meridian and indicate disharmony. Imbalances in the Wood element manifest as headaches, menstrual irregularities, PMS, allergies, digestive problems, stress, or high blood pressure.

In Chinese medicine the organs are believed to have spiritual and emotional properties (in addition to their physiological function). The liver is considered the "planner," while the gallbladder is responsible for making decisions and executing the plans. The liver holds the blueprint of our soul's purpose, enabling us to manifest our unique path without blindly following others. A healthy Wood element will give us the vision and drive to accomplish our goals.

Adaptability is the key to maintaining a balanced Wood element, an element that is easily disrupted by excess emotions. Wood reminds us to be yielding like the willow tree, while remaining strong and grounded within ourselves. Learning to be gentle, compliant, and patient are the lessons of this element.

The yellow-green hue of early spring buds is the healing color for the liver and gallbladder. While doing your Qigong exercises, visualize this radiant light bathing these two organs, rejuvenating your cellular matrix. You can also boost your Wood element by eating green foods full of chlorophyll and life. Think green: collards, kale, Swiss chard, dandelions, wheat grass, and a myriad of salad greens all support healthy liver functioning. If you can't bear to eat them, then get a green powder drink and add it to smoothies. Juice made from fresh greens provides numerious vitamins, minerals, and antioxidants, bringing instant nourishment and energy into your body.

Qigong Attunement: Wood Element

As you begin your Qigong practice, imagine a taproot extending down from the base of your spine (or from your feet) into the ground. Visualize this root slowly winding its way through the dirt, around rocks, through sand and water, until it reaches deep into the Earth. Feel your energy anchored beneath you. Settle your focus into your belly with long, slow breaths. Then gently draw energy up from the Earth through your feet into the lower *dantian*. This Earthly Qi will center you if you are scattered, anxious, or too mentally fixated. It will also nourish the quiet yin and feminine qualities of your being.

Qigong Tree Stance

I usually do my Qigong in a beautiful park with magnificent trees. The Chinese believe the evergreens, particularly pine trees, emit the most Qi, which is further amplified if you're in the mountains. Go to a tree that you're attracted to and stand by it. Get in the Hugging the Tree Pose (see chapter 5, Stances, p. 30). Create a circle with your arms as if you were embracing the aura of the tree and imagine merging with the Qi field of the tree to fortify your own energy. You can also angle your palms toward the roots or up to the branches as you feel led. Each species has its own unique quality. A Taoist Qigong master taught me to use the Qi of Nature to supplement and build my own healing force, so I stand with oaks when I need strength and pines when I need comfort. Experiment with different trees and become acquainted with their diverse energies. After this exchange of energy, I bless the tree and thank it for nourishing me.

FIRE ELEMENT

Organ Systems:	Heart and Small Intestine, plus the Pericardium and Triple Heater Meridians
Color:	Red
Emotion:	Joy vs. Anxiety, Stress
Season:	Summer
Direction:	South
Hours:	Heart 11 A.M.–1 P.M.; Small Intestine 1–3 P.M.; Pericardium 7–9 P.M.; Triple Heater 9–11 P.M.
Taste:	Bitter
Sensory Organ:	Tongue (Speech)

The Nature of Fire

Fire is the spark of life, the warmth of the sun, the heat of a flame. Summer is the season of Fire, when everything is flourishing, blooming, and maturing. The seeds sown in the Wood time of spring come into fruition and are at their zenith in the Fire of summer. It is the most yang-influenced, active time in the cycle, with abundant growth, joyful activities, and transformation. Fire provides us with the warmth, comfort, and radiant light that sustain our life on Earth.

The organs associated with Fire are the heart and small intestine and the meridians of the triple heater and pericardium. The heart is the supreme ruler of the body and regulates the rhythm of our life, balancing the body, mind, and spirit. Not only does the heart oversee blood pressure and circulation, but it is also responsible for our intuitive insight, spiritual connection, and compassion. Its companion organ, the small intestine, regulates digestion and the assimilation of nutrition, separating the pure from the impure. This action not only pertains to food but also our thoughts, beliefs, and actions.

The pericardium is the shock absorber for the heart, deflecting the emotional glitches and traumas of daily life and relationships. This is the meridian acupuncturists treat for heartache, loss, stress, and imbalanced *Shen* (spirit) to help keep the heart intact and functioning without disturbance. The triple heater meridian regulates the warmth and temperature throughout the body and is often referred to as an envelope protecting the organs and regulating immunity. When any of these systems is out of alignment, a person may experience anxiety, insomnia, stress or mental disorders, as well as digestive and cardiac complaints.

Joy and passion are the uplifting feelings of the heart, whereas anxiety, sorrow, and stress can weaken the system. Even excess joy can make a person scattered and unaware of her surroundings. A healthy Fire element bestows us with vitality, stamina, and the ability to follow our passions and complete projects. Our spirit radiates through our eyes and our hearts are open to all of life.

Eating bitter foods (such as dandelions, endive, and escarole) strengthens the heart. This is not a common flavor in our sugar-laden diets, but it is often seen in other countries in the form of digestive bitters after a meal. Classic Chinese foods to nourish the Fire are millet, lamb, plums, and green leafy vegetables; although in summer it's best to eat plenty of fresh fruit and vegetables that are juicy and succulent, along with drinking energizing water.

Qigong Attunement: Fire Element

While practicing Qigong, take the time to slow down and breathe in joy while letting go of anxiety and stress. Attune to your breathing and imagine love filling your heart with a rosy hue (the healing color of the Fire element). Initiate a spontaneous, formless Qigong, performing whatever movements emerge. Allow the slow rhythm to guide you into relaxation and serenity. Let go of time, plans, and structure, and bring yourself into a deeper surrender to the moment. This is great medicine for the heart.

Sun Absorption

Lie on your back in the sun with your knees splayed open and the soles of your feet touching each other. Stretch your arms overhead with palms together. Breathe deeply into your abdomen as you absorb the heat and light waves into your body. This will increase the yang energy to boost your vitality. You can also imagine breathing up and down the central channel of your body by inhaling up through your vagina to the top of your head and down again. This visualization is very energizing and stimulating, clearing your chakras as it reawakens any latent sensuality.

EARTH ELEMENT

Organ Systems:	Spleen (Pancreas) and Stomach
Color:	Yellow
Emotion:	Contentment vs. Worry, Overthinking
Season:	Indian Summer
Direction:	Middle
Hours:	Spleen 9–11 A.M.; Stomach 7–9 A.M.
Taste:	Sweet
Sensory Organ:	Mouth (Taste)

The Nature of Earth

The Earth is the ground upon which we stand, the source of our food and nourishment, the place we call home. We are born of this element and it is the place we will return: it encompasses both the womb and tomb. She is our mother, round and life-supporting, symbolizing fecundity, sensuality, and the rhythms of life. Earth is the center of all the elements from which life arises. A strong Earth gives us stability and allows us to feel connected to the world while maintaining an inner focus. She provides a center to balance our lives with order and harmony.

The digestive organs (the Chinese consider the pancreas as part of the spleen system) are associated with the Earth. In Chinese medicine the stomach and spleen are the providers of postnatal Qi (energy derived from food/drink) that sustains us after birth. The stomach over-sees decomposition of food through digestion and then passes the nutrients on to the spleen to distribute throughout the body. The spleen also controls the muscles, makes blood, and holds the organs in place.

Common Earth imbalances are expressed as digestive problems, addictions, fatigue, infertility, weight challenges, allergies, and chronic immune disorders. Disharmonies may affect the rhythm of our cycles such as menstrual irregularities, disturbed sleep, and bioclock imbalances from travel and working at odd hours.

Dampness impairs the function of the spleen, causing mucous, vaginal discharge, loose stools, bloating, and a sensation of heaviness in the lower body. This can occur from both internal and environmental sources. Women are especially susceptible during menstruation or after childbirth. Situations that could cause dampness are sitting around in a wet bathing suit, living on the coast or in foggy areas, or consuming excessive sugar and dairy products. Candida is a typical damp spleen problem resulting from a poor diet.

Worry, overanalysis, and intense study all adversely affect the Earth energy. A woman with a weakened Earth element may feel uprooted, uncoordinated, nervous, spacey, or insecure. I find many women, especially healers, have difficulty receiving love and support, yet they are impeccable in their ability to supply it to others. This is the classic sign of an imbalanced Earth element. The ability to receive support and nourishment and to live with compassion and empathy are characteristics of a strong and grounded Earth element.

Yellow and orange foods (such as squash, yams, carrots, and millet) support a healthy

Earth element. Eat warming foods (both in temperature and quality) like meat, ginger, and curry spices. Avoid cold foods, such as excess salads, and sweets. As much as possible eliminate sugar from your diet by substituting fresh seasonal fruits grown locally. Get in the habit of drinking water without ice to promote digestion. As the famous nutritionist Bernard Jenson advised, "Eat a rainbow"—fresh, vibrant, and alive foods. We truly are what we eat, so fill yourself with color and light to honor the sacred temple of your body.

Qigong Attunement: Earth Element

Go to a field or garden to practice Qigong and smell the Earth beneath you. Practicing barefoot is especially beneficial if you are a caregiver or if you have a tendency to be scattered. Stand in the Basic Qigong Stance and hold your palms toward the ground, arms hanging loosely by your sides. Breathe in the yin (mother essence of Earth) and draw it up through your feet, legs, and pelvis to settle into your belly (*dantian*), nourishing and replenishing your core power. Remain in this meditative posture for three to ten minutes.

As you stand in this position, visualize golden light (the healing color of the Earth) filling your being, radiating outward from your belly like the sun. Surround your body with a golden orb, creating your own inner sanctuary of safety and peace.

If you're feeling particularly unsettled, then you can "ground" yourself by gardening or lying down outside in nature. Being connected with the Earth will always nurture you, especially during busy or stressful times.

METAL ELEMENT

Organ Systems:	Lungs and Large Intestine
Color:	White
Emotion:	Sadness, Grief vs. Courage
Season:	Autumn
Direction:	West
Hours:	Lungs 3–5 A.M.; Large Intestine 5–7 A.M.
Taste:	Spicy
Sensory Organ:	Nose (Smell)

The Nature of Metal

How do we experience Metal in Nature and within ourselves? Ores are mined from the Earth and welded into structures; crystals are polished into gems that are used in crystal healing or incorporated into communication networks. Metal forms the structure of our society: buildings and vast networks of transportation allow for the flow of telecommunications throughout the world.

Physically, minerals give our body strength, build our internal skeletal structure, and nourish our nervous system. They aid the communication of the nerve synapses and cellular structure throughout the body, as well as support a multitude of body functions. Around the world, healing mineral baths are sought to purify toxicity and provide deep relaxation and release.

In Chinese medicine, autumn corresponds to the Metal element and the organ systems of the lungs and large intestine. During the fall, as the leaves change color and drop to the ground, it is not uncommon to experience sadness, the emotion associated with the lungs. The Metal element also governs the ability to let go (large intestine) and includes the willingness to release physical and emotional wastes (including outdated beliefs). Being consumed by sadness and grief will weaken the lungs and holding on to the past will affect the colon.

At the core of many lung and colon ailments is unresolved grief, often from childhood, that needs to be cleared. Imbalances in these systems can lead to constipation, diarrhea, headache, lung disorders, sinus congestion, allergies, irritability, fatigue, and a loss of enthusiasm for life. The positive emotions of a strong Metal element are courage and righteousness, enabling you to harvest your own gifts and share them with the world. "Inspire" the universal energies and be grateful for each precious breath of life!

In autumn the surface heat of the body begins to move inward, so it's important to dress warmly and protect yourself (especially your neck and head) from the winds. Similarly, you must prepare your body internally during this time of encroaching coolness. Emphasize warmer foods such as grains, legumes, root vegetables, and dark leafy greens to build your body's energy reserve for winter. Reduce your intake of the cooling foods of summer, such as sweet fruits, juice, and salads.

Excessive dryness injures the lungs, so if you live in an arid climate or are affected by internal dryness with flaky skin, dull hair, itchiness, skin problems, or hard stool, then concentrate on drinking more water and eating moistening foods, such as soybean products, barley, millet, spinach, pears, apples, seaweed, shellfish, and eggs.

The lungs and colon are particularly sensitive to poor eating habits and a sedentary lifestyle. Overeating, ingesting too much meat, dairy, and processed meals, or smoking cigarettes can all create excess mucous, clogging up these organs of elimination. Eat a varied diet, balance exercise with quiet contemplative practices, and allow the process of life to move through you with ease and grace.

Qigong Attunement: Metal Element

To experience the energy of the Metal element, practice the Lung Healing Sound exercise in the midst of rocks or boulders, facing your body to the west. Concentrate on breathing in the healing energies of the Universe and imagine filling your whole body with white light. As you exhale, release any sadness, depression, or toxins from your body. Allow your entire being to be filled with energy and radiant light. (See chapter 8, p. 51 for a full description).

Many patients wake up with a dry cough during the early morning lung hours from 3:00 to 5:00 A.M. This indicates that the lungs are energetically weak and need bolstering, so early morning Qigong would be a good remedy to get the Metal element back into alignment. You don't have to get up at that hour, but start your day with Qigong and see how much better you feel throughout your day.

Another way to attune to Metal is to sit and meditate with a crystal or chant along with the tone of a crystal singing bowl. The crystal energy is subtle but can restructure your energetic body so you feel refreshed with an expanded consciousness.

WATER ELEMENT

Organ Systems:	Kidneys and Urinary Bladder
Color:	Blue-Black, Black
Emotion:	Fear vs. Trust, Faith
Season:	Winter
Direction:	North
Hours:	Bladder 3–5 P.M.; Kidneys 5–7 P.M.
Taste:	Salty
Sensory Organ:	Ears (Hearing)

The Nature of Water

Water is movement and tides, waterfalls and lakes, rivulets and oceans, still and stormy. It carves out landscapes over millennia or inundates areas within minutes. It's affected by the moon, sun, wind, and Earth. This planet depends on water to sustain life and we are intimately connected to the energy of Water, since our bodies are composed of more than 75 percent water.

The Water element controls the fluids in the body, including blood, lymph, hormones, and secretions. It is associated with the kidneys (including the adrenals) and urinary bladder. The kidneys govern the skeleton, brain, and reproductive and regenerative properties of the body. When there is an imbalance within this element, we may experience brittle bones; low-back or knee pain; urinary, reproductive, or cardiac dysfunction; as well as premature aging.

Water teaches us to release fear and go with the flow of life. People with a weak Water element often lose their willpower/ambition and are more prone to depression. They may have weak boundaries and are easily pushed around by others. Fear is the emotion that rules the Water element, and it tends to manifest more as women enter perimenopause and menopause. During this change kidney energy wanes and more anxieties surface, often revealing issues that have been buried for decades. It is helpful to strengthen this element before the onset of perimenopause, so your emotions can remain as still as a mountain lake during this transformation.

Winter is the season of Water, so it is important to eat what are considered "warming" and "nourishing" foods to restore your essence. Traditional foods to boost the kidneys are black and adzuki beans, dates, beans/peas, pork, leeks, and fish. Drink herbal tonics like ginseng or Shou Wu Chih, available in Chinese grocery and herb stores.

By learning to honor the natural tides of life, our energy will flow smoothly, traveling around obstacles with ease and grace. Water supports both movement and stillness, reminding us to surrender and trust our deepest knowing. Being able to adapt, activate our willpower, and live gracefully are benefits of a strong Water element.

Qigong Attunement: Water Element

There is a reason why fountains have become so popular: rivers, oceans, and waterfalls are calming and cleansing, and they provide powerful energies for healing. If you live by water, practice Qigong there to bathe and cleanse your energy field. Waterfalls are the most invigorating and will lift your spirit and enliven your Qi. The ocean is expansive and meditative, inviting you to attune to the primordial essence of your being (try the Sea Meditation described in chapter 6, p. 35). Explore the different manifestations of Water and release your fears as you sink into a harmonious inner flow.

If you reach for caffeine or sugar in the afternoons, instead of grabbing a latte, practice the Dragon Spiraling up the Pillar exercise (see chapter 17, Insomnia, p. 122) along with the Lymph Pump (chapter 14, Breast Health, p. 100) to reactivate your energy. This is also a great time to do your Qigong routine, releasing stressors from the day and bringing in new Qi for the evening. I find it very balancing and tend to sleep better at night.

The Five Elements teach us about our inseparable connection with Nature. The Chinese understood that the one inherent truth in life is that change is inevitable. As the monk Thich Nhat Hanh reflected, "Keeping your body healthy is an expression of gratitude to the whole cosmos—the trees, the clouds, everything."[1] If we learn to adapt our lifestyle to the seasonal fluctuations, then we may live in balance and harmony within ourselves and be mutually supported by our environment.

8

Six Healing Sounds

The natural healing force within each of us
is the greatest force in getting well.

—Hippocrates

THE SIX HEALING SOUNDS are resonances that were formulated by the ancient Chinese to regulate and heal the organ systems. Tao Hongjing (456–536 C.E.), a famous Chinese doctor, compiled this ancient knowledge, which later became popularized in contemporary China by the revered Qigong master and traditional Chinese doctor Ma Litang.

The Six Healing Sounds dispel toxic energy and improve organ function, promoting health for the entire body. Illness appears on an energetic level prior to manifesting in the body, so these exercises can be used to clear emotional and physical blocks (that affect organ function)

to help prevent disease. Toning them will bring you into a deeper appreciation and awareness of the remarkable inner alchemy of your body. (Listen to the sounds on my Web site, www.womensqigong.com.)

When you do these exercises, old emotions, feelings, and memories may percolate up, finding their way into your dreams, or as fleeting images and moods throughout the day. Pay attention to what emerges as you begin voicing the healing sounds. Since your body holds cellular memories, intoning and feeling the resonance of these sounds will enable you to release and heal old patterns. Be open to the possibility of subtle yet profound healing.

49

UNDERSTANDING THE SIX HEALING SOUNDS

Every yin organ (lungs, kidneys, liver, heart, spleen) plus the triple heater meridian has a healing sound. While each sound affects its specific organ(s), it also aids the corresponding yang organ. For example, by doing the lung healing sound you will also be influencing the large intestine. The Six Healing Sounds exercises are included in many of the Qigong protocols in this book; they can also be done as a separate practice to regulate your organ health and keep your system balanced. (See fig. 8.1.)

Each healing sound sequence is to be done in sets of six. Perform the sounds in accordance with the flow of the Five Element chart. I usually begin with the lung exercise, follow with kidney, liver, heart, and triple heater, and end with spleen. If you're weak in one area, do the exercise for that organ for two to three sets with a few relaxing breaths in between intervals. Be sure to hold the exhalation for a prolonged period while intoning the healing sounds to augment the detoxifying benefits, even if they may seem awkward to perform at first.

After completing each sequence, take a few minutes to gently smile down to each organ, thanking your body for keeping you healthy and alive. Smiling has been proven to boost the

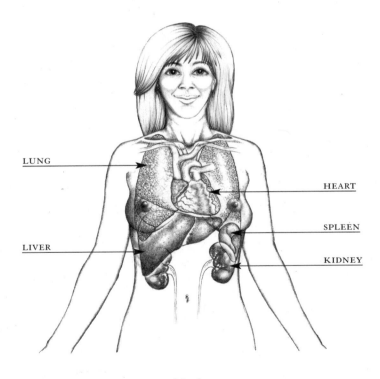

LUNG

HEART

SPLEEN

LIVER

KIDNEY

[8.1]

immune system, so allow it to be a genuine smile emerging from your heart. Imagine the energy and light that your smile radiates, and shine that inwardly toward your organs with sincere gratitude and love.

Following you will find an explanation of each of the Six Healing Sounds.

LUNG

I've witnessed the immediate impact of these exercises repeatedly. At a weeklong retreat in Santa Barbara, I was teaching the first in a series of classes in Qigong. I usually don't expect much from the first class since people are just getting settled from traveling. During this particular class, while practicing the lung exercise, I could see a man quietly crying. After class, I asked what he was experiencing, and he began sobbing. He had just lost his dog and hadn't been able to cry about it yet. While clutching his chest, he shared that the Qigong opened the gate to his tears, facilitating a great release. By the end of the retreat, he felt the Qigong helped him process the death and come to peace within his heart.

The emotions associated with the lungs are sadness and grief. Its companion organ, the large intestine, controls the letting go of both body waste and beliefs that no longer serve us. When you exhale, imagine releasing emotions or ideas that dampen your vitality. On the inhalation, bring in the healing energies of the Universe, showering each cell with vitality and white light (the healing color of the lungs). Breathe in courage and fortify your body with strength.

These sounds will be described phonetically and they should be quietly pronounced on the exhalations.

Lung Healing Sound: Sh-ay

During the exhalation, sound "sh" until the very end of your exhalation then add the sound "ay" (as though you were saying the word "shade" without the "d" on the end). This resonance strengthens the lungs, expels excess mucous and toxins, and releases grief and sadness. The lung exercise will help heal asthma, emphysema, allergies, and any lung condition.

1. Stand in the Basic Qigong Stance.
Inhale
2. Draw a circle with your hands by lifting your arms laterally with palms facing upward, until your hands come together with palms touching above your head.
3. Lower your hands along the front midline to meet in prayer position at your heart, with your palms together and your elbows horizontal to the ground.
Exhale
4. Open your palms outward and rotate to the side (as though you were opening a book so it faces away from your body), simultaneously drop your elbows to press gently against your ribs, and continue turning your hands and arms so your forearms and palms are facing away from your body.
5. Press out to your sides with hands flexed at the wrists until your arms are extended fully (as if you're pushing away two walls that are closing in on you).
6. Then relax your arms at your sides.

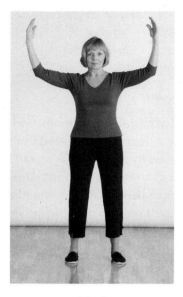
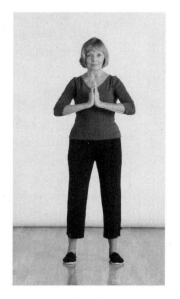
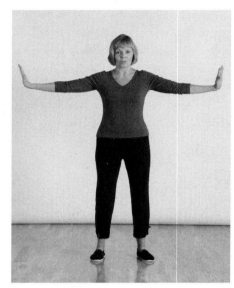

[8.2]   [8.3]   [8.4]

Inhale while raising your arms to prayer position.

Exhale while pushing out to the sides. Time the completion of your exhalation to coincide with your arms being fully extended. Relax your arms so they hang down by your sides before inhaling again.

Repeat the entire cycle of movements six times. (See figs. 8.2, 8.3, and 8.4.)

KIDNEY

The kidneys support graceful aging, strong bones, and mental acuity so it's important to include kidney Qigong into your daily routine. Fear diminishes the resiliency of the Water element so release your fears on the exhalation and bring in trust or faith with each breath.

Kidney Healing Sound: Chu-ay

To make the sound "chu" (like "chew"), round your lips with your tongue behind the teeth and slightly raised. The second half of the resonance is voiced as a long "a." The healing sound for the kidneys is beneficial for urinary and cardiac problems, bone/spinal strength, brain health, hearing, reproductive diseases, and any age-related issues, as well as to support overall health and longevity.

Stand a little wider than the Basic Qigong Stance. Place your palms against your lower back and inhale while bringing them upward to your lower ribs warming your lower back and kidney/adrenal area.

1. Exhale as you move your palms back down. Repeat three times.

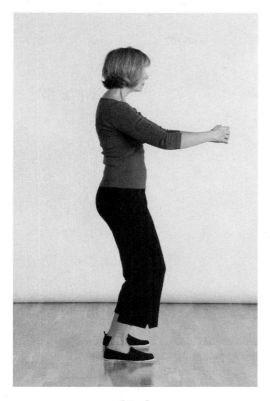

[8.5]

Inhale

2. Again bring your hands up to your kidney area.

Exhale

3. Quietly say "chu-ay" as you squat comfortably down while circling your arms out in front as if holding a beach ball. Knees should not extend past your toes. Relax your shoulders and hold your arms level with your chest. Try to remain centered without leaning forward too much.

4. At the end of your exhalation, stand up into Basic Qigong Stance with arms by your sides. Repeat the whole sequence three or six times. (See fig. 8.5.)

LIVER

The liver meridian controls the smooth flow of Qi throughout the body, so if you are stressed, there will be an imbalance here. This usually manifests as anger, frustration, depression, edginess, and a host of physical ailments such as PMS and menstrual irregularities. If you tend to be moody, include this healing sound in your daily program.

Liver Healing Sound: Shuu *("shoe")*

The liver sound "Shuu" is pronounced like "shoe." The emphasis is on the "sh" for most of the exhalation and then the "uu" is included at the end. With each prolonged exhalation, imagine letting go of your stress, painful emotions, or any feelings of being stuck in your life. This healing sound relieves congestion in the liver meridian and is beneficial for many conditions such as emotional upset, depression, allergies, indigestion, fatigue, hypertension, and anxiety.

1. Stand in the Basic Qigong Stance. Place the backs of your hands together (wrist to wrist, with the fingers facing down as though they are in a backward and upside-down prayer position) along the midline of your lower abdomen.

Inhale

No movement.

Exhale

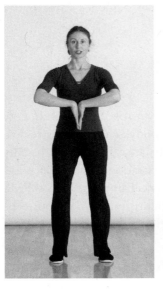

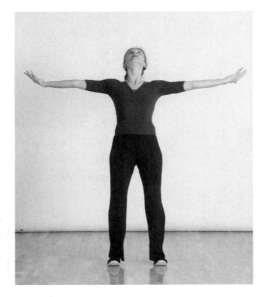

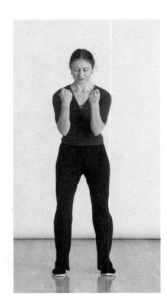

[8.6]   [8.7]   [8.8]

2. Raise your hands up the midline of your body to chest level, and continue the movement so your arms are like a fountain spraying open above your head.

3. Rock back on your heels as you open your arms outward, stretching your arms out to your sides so your face and palms are facing the heavens.

4. Open your chest to the sky.

5. Continue by rocking forward into regular stance as you circle your arms forward at shoulder level with palms and forearms outstretched as if holding a tray.

6. Then fold your forearms and your fists into your chest, lean slightly forward as you squeeze any stagnancy or stale air out of the torso.

7. Remember to voice "shuu" for the entire exhalation. Release! Open up your arms to

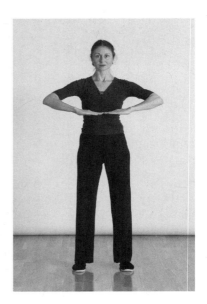

[8.9]

circulate new Qi throughout your mind-body and affirm: *"I am relaxed and flexible in my life. I am resilient!"* (See figs. 8.6, 8.7, and 8.8.)

Inhale

8. Open your fists and turn your open palms toward the ground. Your forearms should be parallel to the ground with your fingertips almost touching in front of your chest. Press down the midline with a full inhalation. This final move is also repeated in the heart healing sound movement. (See fig. 8.9)

Repeat this series for a total of six repetitions.

HEART

The heart exercise is particularly beneficial for menopausal women and others challenged by insomnia. Women in my menopause classes experience quick results by doing both the Heart and Triple Heater Healing Sounds. Perform one to two sets (six to twelve repetitions) of each before bed to promote sleep.

Heart Healing Sound: Huuh

The healing sound "huuh" is guttural and you'll feel it in your throat. This sound is similar to a guttural pronunciation of the word "hook" without the "k" on the end.

You can use this exercise for all heart conditions, anxiety, insomnia, depression, restlessness, fatigue, and stress.

1. Stand in the Basic Qigong Stance. Place your hands on your lower abdomen with your palms face up; your fingers should almost be touching, creating a circle with your arms.

Inhale

No movement.

Exhale

2. Raise your hands to heart level; keep your palms flat and arms formed in an oval shape.

3. Turn your palms outward as you bring your hands up to your temples with your thumbs next to your temples. Look upward.

4. Then rotate your hands inward, with palms a few inches in front of your eyes and emit soothing Qi into your eyes. Close your eyes for a moment in relaxation.

5. Slowly lower your hands to heart level while reopening your eyes. Your hands and forearms should be about a fist's width away from your body.

Inhale

6. Turn your palms toward the ground with fingers almost touching (as in the liver exercise) and push your hands and arms down as you inhale.

Repeat the whole sequence six times. (See figs. 8.10, 8.11, and 8.12 that follow.)

TRIPLE HEATER

The triple heater (also called "triple burner" or "sanjiao") is a meridian that regulates the temperature of the three zones of the body: the upper heater controls the upper torso, including the heart and lungs; the middle heater oversees the digestive organs, including the stomach and spleen; the lower heater includes

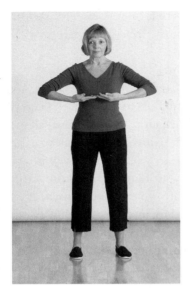 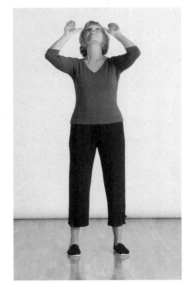 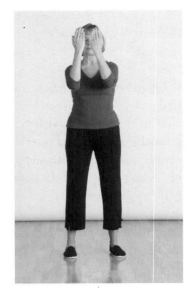

[8.10]   [8.11]   [8.12]

the kidneys, intestines, and bladder. Balancing this energy system is particularly helpful in managing the symptoms of menopause.

Triple Heater Healing Sound: Sss

The healing resonance for the triple heater is "*sss*." While exhaling, point the tip of your tongue downward and pull your mouth back, slightly raising the corners of your mouth, as if smiling. The Triple Heater Sound will help relieve insomnia, hot flashes, night sweats, and anxiety by regulating the temperature throughout your body and relieving excess heat and agitation.

1. Stand in Basic Qigong Stance with your arms at your sides.

Inhale

2. Bring your arms into a circle along the midline of your lower belly; your middle fingers will almost be touching and your palms will be flat and facing upward. Hold your hands a few inches from your body.

Exhale

3. Slowly raise your hands up the center of your torso (fingers almost touching) and stop right below your chin. Keep your palms and forearms flat (parallel with the ground) with your elbows extended out to the sides.

4. Rotate and raise your hands out in front of you so they're above your head with your palms facing outward. Your hands are separated and about shoulder-width apart (as though you're being held up by a bank robber). Look upward.

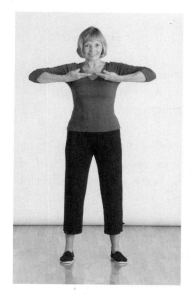 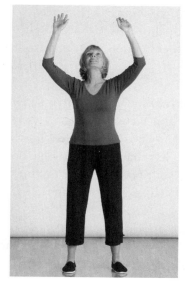 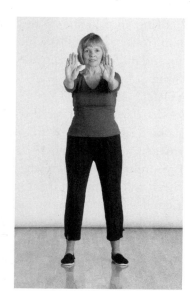

[8.13]   [8.14]   [8.15]

5. Keeping your arms in front of you, slowly lower your hands to heart level, with your palms facing outward, then press forward.

6. Your exhalation should end when your arms are fully extended in front and your hands are flexed.

Inhale

7. Inhale as you bring your arms back to your sides.

Complete six rounds. (See figs. 8.13, 8.14, and 8.15.)

SPLEEN

The spleen regulates digestion, produces blood, and controls the blood sugar levels in the body; therefore this exercise is essential for women with diabetes, hypoglycemia, or digestive disorders.

Spleen Healing Sound: Hoo

The healing sound for the spleen (pancreas) is "hoo," which is similar to the sound of the wind or blowing out a candle. While exhaling, release all worries and overthinking (which weakens the spleen energy) and infuse yourself with contentment and peacefulness. This movement will help with all digestive problems, bloating, diarrhea, fatigue, worry, and chronic illness.

I. Stand in Basic Qigong Stance.
Inhale

2. Bring your hands up to your diaphragm area (in front of your ribs) with your palms facing up and fingertips facing one another but not touching.

Exhale

3. Move your right hand to the midline of your outer right thigh, with your palm facing downward, and your fingers pointing forward.

4. Simultaneously, stretch your left hand overhead and slightly in front of the your body; your hand is flexed, palm up, fingers point back over your head.

5. Twist at the waist to the right and look behind you.

Inhale

6. Bend your knees as you return to center, facing front.

7. Simultaneously move your palms to the midline (left hand by heart and right hand by lower abdomen), facing one another as if holding a vessel.

8. Slowly bring them together (moving the left one down and the right one up) along the midline of the body, until they meet in the center.

Exhale

9. Twist to the left and stretch upward as before but now with your left palm down by

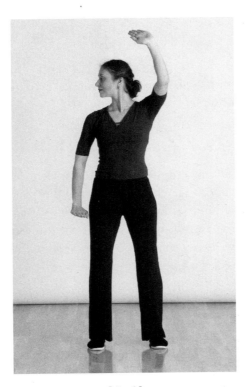

[8.16]

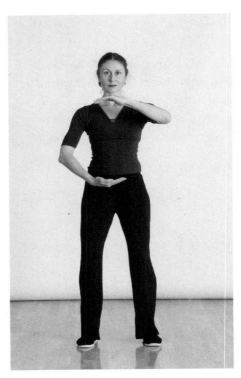

[8.17]

your thigh and your right hand overhead. As you twist, look back over your left shoulder.

10. Return to the center as before but with your right hand on top and your left on the bottom; knees are bent. This is a continual movement as you again switch hand positions and twist to the right.

On each exhalation, say "hoo" like you're gently blowing out a candle. Repeat the sequence six times to each side. (See figs. 8.16 and 8.17.)

PART TWO

Healthy, Fit, and Sexy at Any Age

9

Dynamic Woman

AGES FORTY TO
FORTY-NINE

THIS IS THE TIME in a woman's life that is full of opportunity, zest, and abundance. When healthy, a young woman's Qi is vital and her body is resilient, with enough energy to raise a family and follow her career. Unfortunately, with seemingly limitless reserves, many women take on too much, juggling kids and work (and husbands). Consumed by commitments, women often don't take enough time for themselves, their needs plummet to the bottom of the priority list, and their health may suffer from this neglect.

The most active time in the reproductive stage of a woman's life is during her twenties to early forties, so it's imperative to replenish blood lost in menstruation and keep the reproductive organs healthy with sufficient Qi. Many women in their late thirties and forties come to my clinic with complaints of PMS, emotional swings, cramps, or other menstrual

disorders. These problems can be easily alleviated through the practice of Qigong by regulating the flow of Qi and nourishing the liver, spleen, and blood. It's important to begin garnering your energy, especially while you're young and healthy, to maintain your vitality and slow the hormonal decline that occurs in menopause. A consistent Qigong practice can become your lifetime ritual for youthful renewal and self-nurturance.

The Dynamic Woman Qigong program was developed for younger women to build and preserve their overall health, agility, and strength by moving and balancing the Qi in their meridians, strengthening the upper body and legs, and stimulating breast Qi. Unlike other Qigong exercises in this book, these exercises are designed to flow sequentially. For optimal results, a twenty- to thirty-minute program performed daily is best, followed by meditation. Add the breast cancer prevention exercises (chapter 14, Breast Health) to your routine twice a week or daily if you have a history of breast cancer in your family.

Remember: embrace your practice with joy and love and take the time now to maintain and nourish your gift of health.

DYNAMIC WOMAN SERIES OF EXERCISES AND STANCES

This is a complete sequence, with one movement flowing into the next. Begin by performing each of the exercises in multiples of eight, the female number for balance and harmony. As you get stronger you can increase the repetitions.

Dantian *Breathing*

1. Stand in Basic Qigong Stance. Begin by gathering your energy into your *dantian* (below your belly button) with deep abdominal breathing. Place your right hand over your *dantian* and your left hand on top of your right.

2. Make sure your tongue is gently touching the roof of your mouth and contract your anus gently with each exhalation.

3. Focus your attention with each breath into your *dantian*. Feel your feet grounded into Mother Earth, standing firm and strong.

Be still until you feel centered.

Awkward Stance

1. Stand with heels touching and your toes splayed outward, forming a right angle with your feet.

Inhale

2. Lift up on your toes, keep your heels touching each other as you rise.

3. Concurrently draw a large circle with your arms: first raise your arms to the sides and circle them overhead to meet in front of you, just above your head, with palms joining. Slowly lower them to your chest in prayer position.

Exhale

4. Remaining on your toes, squat down and sink into bent knees while continuing to hold your heels together and hands in prayer position.

5. Concentrate on *dantian* breathing. If you have difficulty balancing, look at a fixed point directly ahead of you at eye level or about 6 feet in front of your feet on the ground.

Remain in this stance for twenty-four to sixty-four slow breaths with your eyes half closed. If you really want to cultivate strength, then stay in this position for one to three minutes and gradually build up to ten minutes. (For photo see fig. 5.4, chapter 5, Stances, p. 32.)

Side Step

Inhale

1. Keep your arms in the prayer position in the middle of your chest. From your position on

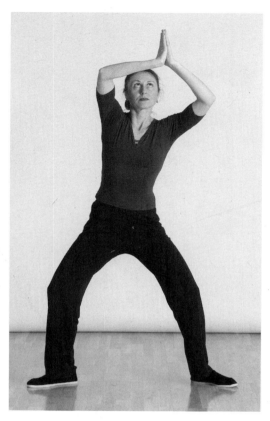

[9.1]

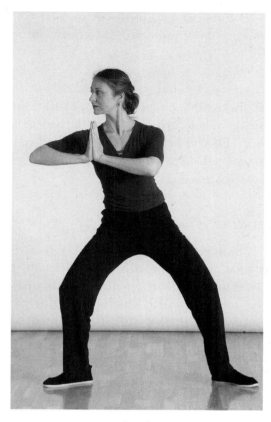

[9.2]

tiptoes, step to the side with your right leg into a Modified Horse Stance (legs 2 to 3 feet apart); plant both feet on the ground.

2. Simultaneously circle your arms (and hands held in prayer position) counterclockwise, crossing in front of your chest, and then raise them above your head. At all times keep your palms pressed together. Complete the circle with your palms coming back into prayer position at heart level.

Exhale

3. Push your right elbow horizontally out to the side (left palm is pushing against right palm); keep your forearms parallel to the ground. As you press your elbow to the right, shift your weight onto the right foot: this magnifies your power. This is a martial arts move, so imagine you're hitting someone with your elbow and use your exhalation to power the strike.

4. Now do the same series of movements in reverse toward the opposite side (clockwise, to

the left): the circling of the palms and elbow strike are one continuous movement on both sides.

By pressing your palms together, you activate the lymph under your arms—the main drainage area for toxins for both the breasts and torso. This will help keep your breasts healthy and uplifted. Repeat eight times on each side. (See figs. 9.1 and 9.2.)

Beautiful Woman Pose

1. Shift your weight onto your left foot, then lift your right thigh so it is parallel with the ground with your toes pointed down, similar to the standing pose of a crane.
2. At the same time stretch your left arm above your head with your fingers spiraling back as if you were picking an apple; keep your palm facing toward you.
3. Flex your right hand and place it beside your outer right thigh, with your palm facing toward the Earth. (See fig. 9.3.)
4. Stand and do deep *dantian* breathing for 8 breaths. Stretch skyward with each exhalation.
5. Slowly change sides. Step onto your right foot, raise your right hand above your head and lift your left thigh until it is parallel to the floor.

All movements are identical but reversed. As you balance here, visualize and affirm to yourself that you're confident, beautiful, powerful, and steadfast.

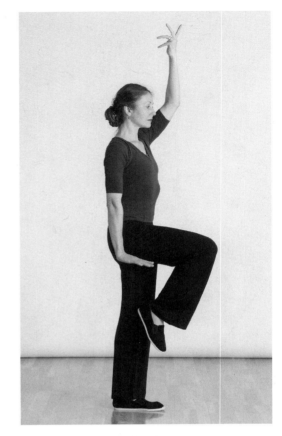

[9.3]

Snake Walk

1. Cross your left leg (that is still lifted in the Beautiful Woman Pose) to step diagonally in front of your right leg at a 45-degree angle.
2. Bend down so the knees of both legs fold close together. At the same time circle your right arm to your chest with your palm straight and facing left, and your fingers pointing to the heavens. Your left arm moves to your midback with palm facing up.

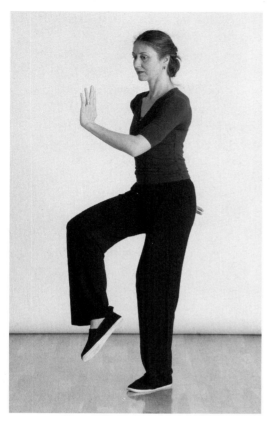

[9.4]

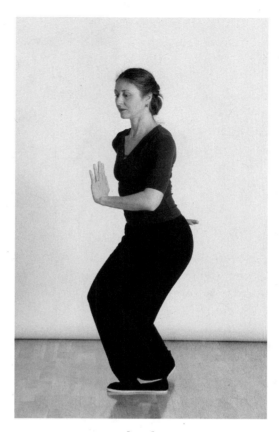

[9.5]

3. Look straight ahead as you walk.

4. Change directions on the next step. This time cross your right leg over the left, while your left palm comes up to your heart area, pointing toward the right. Place your right hand on your midback with the palm facing upward. (See figs. 9.4 and 9.5.)

Squat down as far as you can with each step: make sure you don't strain your knees. The arms move gracefully in semicircles, like a Ba-

linese dancer. Continue for sixteen to thirty-two steps and return to your original starting place.

Arm Wheel

1. Stand in Basic Qigong Stance. Wave your hands in alternating circles out in front of your face circling as low as your pelvis: your right hand goes clockwise while your left moves counterclockwise.

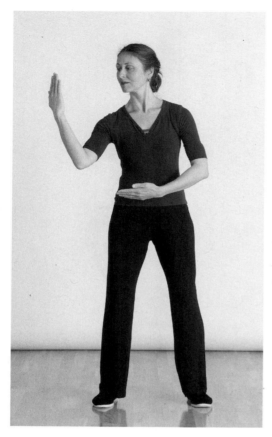

[9.6]

2. One hand is up while the other is down. Your open palm faces you with thumb extended like a mitten. (See fig. 9.6.)

Slowly draw 60 to 120 circles or just continue for a few minutes.

Dunhuang *Meditation*

End this series by standing in *Dunhuang* Meditation (see description in chapter 6, Meditation, p. 36). Stand for twenty-four breaths to calm and regulate your body.

The Dynamic Woman Series blends both upper- and lower-body movements to build stamina, overall body tone, and coordination. These exercises move Qi and blood and activate lymph flow to keep your breasts healthy. You will feel more vitality and balance in your life as you practice this sequence.

SELF-HEALING MASSAGE

Massage is an integral component of Qigong healing both for yourself and others (though this book only includes self-massage). Not only is massage soothing, but it stimulates Qi and blood flow through the organs and meridians. Each massage in this book addresses certain areas or symptoms for healing or preventive care. Include these after your exercises to utilize the Qi you have gathered for self-healing.

Ovary Bridge Massage

1. Lie on your back with the soles of your feet together.

2. Lift your pelvis off the ground so the majority of your weight rests on the sides of your feet and upper back. (See fig. 9.7.)

3. Gently tighten your buttocks and pelvic floor.

4. Place your palms on your lower abdomen right above the inguinal grooves (the creases separating your legs and torso).

5. Massage in small circles sixteen times, or until you feel warmth soothing your abdomen.

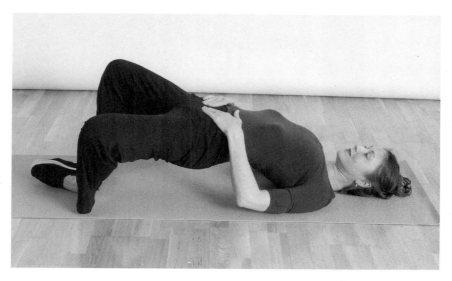

[9.7]

6. Slowly lower down and relax with a few deep belly breaths.

This massage nourishes the ovaries, alleviates congestion in the reproductive organs and meridians, and slows hormonal decline, which begins in perimenopause. Do this daily or at least three times a week.

MEDITATION

Ren Chong *Meditation*

After your Qigong practice, sit for ten minutes and gather your energy into the *ren* and *chong* meridians, which are important in nourishing and regulating the menstrual cycle and will help relieve bloating and digestive issues. (See chapter 6, Meditations, p. 36.)

. You may want to practice Ovary Breathing twice a week to regulate and stimulate your ovaries and reproductive energies. (See chapter 10, Graceful Passage, p. 74.

CONCLUSION

The Dynamic Woman years are the best time to cultivate and store your Qi and blood. By commencing a Qigong routine in your early forties, you will glide through menopause without the uncomfortable hot flashes and night sweats that plague many women. The Dynamic Woman series will empower and support you throughout this most energetic and productive stage of your life.

10

Graceful Passage

PERIMENOPAUSE

THE AGE WHEN a woman enters that transitional phase between *being* the Dynamic Woman and *becoming* the Wise Woman (i.e., moving from a vital, juicy stage of life to the more contemplative energy that comes with menopause) is varied and elusive. It's a passage where we often need to cope with a new identity of ourselves, losing our youthfulness and ability to birth children, yet not yet ready to accept our middle-aged years. Many of us cringe at the thought of our crone years approaching and at the possibility of losing the endless resources of energy that we've always known. Sometimes a woman will go through her change without noticing (though this is rare in our culture), or she may have symptoms for ten years, beginning somewhere between her early forties to fifties. It's prudent to begin a regular Qigong practice at the onset of perimenopause to ensure a gradual hormonal decline and to retain vitality and a balanced emotional state. There are many levels of well-being to navigate during

this passage, so a consistent mind-body practice is extremely beneficial and can allay many complaints.

The focus for the Graceful Passage Qigong is to harmonize your body and mind, calm the emotions, nourish yin, and cultivate your energy. There are a myriad of symptoms that accompany this transitional period, so you may want to augment your routine by adding exercises from the chapters on menopause, PMS, and insomnia, as well as from the Dynamic Woman and Wise Woman programs. Remember to always include the four important components of Qigong healing: (1) gentle movement; (2) a strengthening stance; (3) self-healing massage; and (4) meditation. It's also important to practice the breast cancer prevention exercises twice a week (or daily if breast cancer is common in your family).

This is a significant passage of life that invites us to become more aware of our body and attend to the subtle shifts that are occurring. Change may be uncomfortable, but what will emerge is a new dimension of ourselves as spiritual and creative women.

DYNAMIC EXERCISES

Drinking Essence from Bubbling Spring

This exercise nourishes the kidneys (including the adrenals) and yin fluids of the body (aiding in hormonal and menstrual regulation to reduce fatigue) by drawing energy up through the "Bubbling Spring" points in the soles of your feet.

1. Stand with your feet about 3 feet apart and your knees bent.

2. Place the backs of your hands on the waist area of your back, over the kidneys.

3. Take a few deep breaths and connect with the supportive energy of the Earth below your feet. Visualize and feel the energy point on the soles of both feet, Bubbling Spring (Kidney 1), where the Earth's yin energy enters the body (for point location see fig. 10.1).
Inhale

4. Imagine this essence flowing up from the Earth through your feet, legs, and pelvis to settle into your back, nourishing and revitalizing your kidneys and adrenals.
Exhale

5. Bend your knees as deeply as you can while maintaining a relatively straight back (as if you were about to perch on the edge of a chair). Don't arch your back, as this will strain your lower back and cause your butt to stick out. (See fig. 10.2.)
Inhale

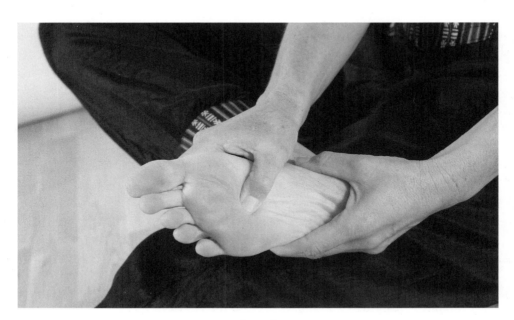

[10.1]

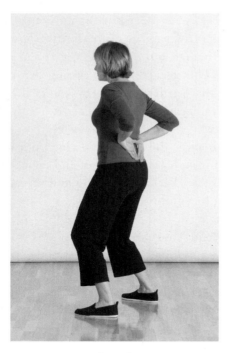

[10.2]

concern. The Japanese call it the "fifty-year shoulder," since tendons and ligaments can become weaker and more easily strained. The Flying Eagle will strengthen the shoulder joint as well as heal shoulder injuries.

1. Stand in Basic Qigong Stance. Lean slightly forward as if you were about to fly (you may also step one foot forward for better balance).

2. Splay your arms out to the sides with your elbows pointing outward and your arms rounded, like you're holding beach balls by your sides. (If you've ever seen raptors, this is how they hold their wings out to dry).

3. Remember to keep your shoulders *down* throughout this exercise to get the most benefit.

4. Place your fingers together and angle them slightly backward. Tuck your chin in slightly.

Inhale

5. Imagine you're flying as you raise your arms to shoulder level, lifting them from the elbows; your arms remain splayed outward (rounded like wings).

6. When you reach shoulder level, extend your hands out so your arms are spread like wings. (See figs. 10.3 and 10.4.)

Exhale

7. Flap your wings downward, pressing down with your upper arms to lend strength to your wings. Imagine you're an eagle with expansive, powerful wings, garnering energies through your flight.

8. As your arms come to about a foot from the sides of your thighs, flip your wrists inward so the palms face upward. Don't actually touch your body.

6. Rise up slowly, drawing energy up from the Earth into the kidneys underneath your hands. Press gently against your back as if you're pulling yourself up while supporting your back.

Exhale as you squat down and *inhale* as you stand. Repeat the squatting/standing routine nine to eighteen times. As you inhale, pull gently upward on your anus to help focus the Qi into your kidneys. This retains the energy in your body without allowing it to leak out.

Flying Eagle

Many women, as they approach fifty, will "mysteriously" get shoulder pain while doing the same activities that they've always done without

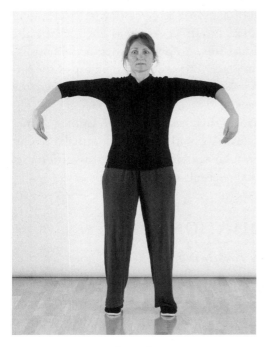

[10.3]

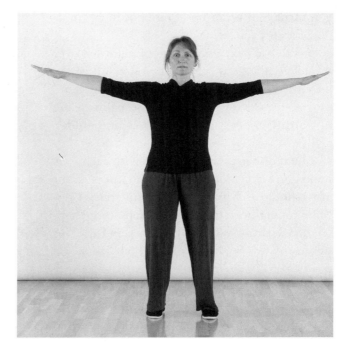

[10.4]

Inhale

9. Angle your hands back again and repeat the flying action, lifting from the elbows.

You should feel this in your upper arms and shoulders. If you have a shoulder injury, then begin with only a few repetitions and gradually increase them as you get stronger. Otherwise, do this exercise nine to eighteen times, or one to two minutes if you are strong. End by loosely flapping your wings to release any tension in the shoulders.

Snake Twist Walk

Walking Qigong strengthens the legs; pumps Qi and blood back into the heart to stimulate cardiovascular health; and develops coordination, grace, and balance.

1. Cross your left leg diagonally in front of your right leg and step out at a 45-degree angle.

2. Bend down so the knees of both legs fold close together.

3. At the same time your right arm circles to your chest with your hand held up, thumb near your breastbone and your palm straight and facing to the left, fingers pointing to the heavens.

4. Your left arm goes to the midback with your palm flat, facing upward.

5. Twist from your waist and look back over your left shoulder. Keep your front hand vertical in alignment with the center of your chest as

you turn; your other hand remains in the middle of your back.

6. On the next step, cross the right leg over the left while your left palm comes up to the heart area, facing the right; your right hand moves toward the back with the palm facing upward. Twist to gaze over your right shoulder.

Squat down as far as you can with each step: make sure you don't strain your knees. Your arms should arch gracefully in semicircles. Continue for eighteen to thirty-six steps. (See chapter 9, Dynamic Woman, figs. 9.4 and 9.5, for photos of the Snake Walk without the twist, p. 67.)

STANCES

Concentrate on practicing either the Three-Circles Stance or Awkward Stance. Remain in the pose for three minutes daily and gradually increase your time to ten to fifteen minutes. Stamina and strength are developed through these stances—the most important vehicle for increasing your immunity and vitality.

SELF-HEALING MASSAGE

Large Intestine Massage

This colon massage is excellent for relieving constipation, bloating, and digestive distress.

Lie down or stand; place your middle three fingers on the lower right corner of your abdomen by the hip. Use firm pressure as you rub your abdomen in a large clockwise circle along your large intestine, which is enclosed by the ribs on the top and pelvic bones at the bottom. You can place your other hand on top of the fingers to add more pressure and stimulation to the intestines.

Perform this massage nine to eighteen times and then relax with deep abdominal breaths. This circular rubbing stimulates digestion and intestinal peristalsis for regularity.

MEDITATION

Ovary Breathing

This concentrated breathing regulates hormones and energizes the sexual system. It's advisable to start gathering Qi into the ovaries in your early forties to build up sufficient energy reserves to ensure a graceful menopause. This is also helpful in healing reproductive issues such as menstrual irregularity and cramps.

Sit on the edge of a firm, level chair with both feet flat on the ground and your back straight. As you sit, adjust your body weight onto your perineum (located halfway between the anus and vagina). To acquaint yourself with this area, you may want to press gently with your fingers, attuning to sensations there. During the breathing, concentrate on the perineum as you pull up gently on the vagina, perineum, and anus.

Inhale deeply as you flex the pelvic floor
Exhale
Do eight short, dynamic exhalations through the nose with an emphasis on pushing the Qi

down to the perineum in short puffs, while simultaneously pulling gently up on your pelvic floor. If you're doing this correctly, your perineum will expand with each exhalation. This breathing should not be forced.

After eight exhalations, focus the energy by inhaling and drawing the Qi up to the Uterine Palace. Hold your breath a few moments to energize this feminine energy center. Take a few relaxing breaths and then begin the sequence again. Remember to keep your anus slightly contracted throughout the exercise and relax your shoulders. Practice the sequence in increments of eight (up to sixty-four times). Add Ovary Breathing two to three times a week to your Qigong routine.

Ren Chong *Meditation*

After your Qigong practice, perform the *Ren Chong* Meditation for ten minutes (for a full description refer to chapter 6, Meditations, p. 36).

ADDITIONAL HEALING AIDS

Include Ovary Bridge Massage (found in chapter 9, Dynamic Woman, p. 68) to stimulate your ovaries and slow the decrease of your hormonal levels.

Push the Mountain will give you more vitality and stabilize emotions, especially anger and depression. (See chapter 13, PMS, p. 93.)

CONCLUSION

In many cultures around the world perimenopause is not even a concept. Most non-American women are usually more physically active in their daily routines and have plant-based diets, both of which are conducive to an easy transition through menopause. By commencing a Qigong routine in your early forties, you can balance your hormones and avoid the uncomfortable symptoms that often define this passage. A regular practice helps ground your energies and stabilize your emotions (which tend to get scattered in perimenopause). Be creative with your routine and make it enjoyable so you will feel empowered as you enter middle age.

11

Wise Woman

AGES FIFTY TO
SIXTY-FOUR

WITH AGE COMES wisdom. A woman entering her fifties is wise to commit to taking care of herself. As we get older, it's harder to gain strength and build bone, so it's important to maintain your physique for a resilient life into the future. Keeping active, breathing deeply, and resting when your body needs restoration are essential components to healthy aging. During the Wise Woman years, many women are frustrated because they can't do what they used to do. Their joints become stiffer and many of my students have turned to Qigong when practicing yoga became too painful or caused injuries. Although how we age is influenced by many factors, such as genetics, lifestyle, stress, and environment (some of which are out of our control), we do have control of how we nurture our bodies on a daily basis.

In midlife, digestion begins to slow and our joints, tendons, and ligaments need more atten-tion and care—a woman's yin (her nurturing fluids) is waning. Wise Woman Qigong primar-ily focuses on strengthening the kidneys to maintain strong bones and a clear mind, as well as nourish the yin that becomes depleted in menopause. The kidneys influence the aging process throughout our lives, so keeping them healthy and balanced is the recipe for longevity.

DYNAMIC EXERCISES

Warm-ups

Do some simple joint rotations to keep you flexible. For example, successively rotate your wrists, shoulders, knees, and ankles along with some slow neck stretches. Be gentle, especially in the morning when your body tends to be stiffer. (To explore additional warm-ups, please refer to chapter 4, Activating Your Energy.)

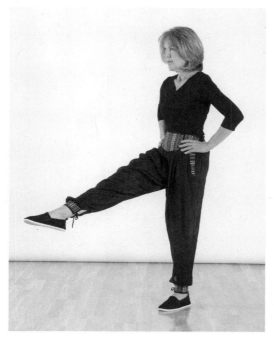

[11.1]

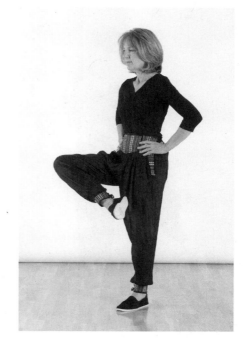

[11.2]

Four-Sided Knee Kick

These multiple kicks strengthen the knee ligaments to stabilize the joint and are helpful for
warming up before running or performing aerobic activities. Begin in Basic Qigong Stance and
either rest your hands on your waist or by your
side. Kick out gently in each direction, allowing
the Qi to activate your legs, not using brute
force. For all of these kicks you can breathe naturally or exhale with each kick outward.

CRANE KICK

Raise your right thigh so it's horizontal to the
ground. Gently kick your right foot out with

your toes pointed, keeping your thigh lifted.
The kick comes from your knee as though
moving a hinge. Lower your foot back to the
ground. Then lift your left leg and kick out
again from your knee. Do this action once on
each side. (See fig. 11.1.)

HALF-LOTUS KICK

Cock and lift your right foot in front of your
body as if preparing to sit in a cross-legged position. Move as though you were going to kick
your left thigh with the inside arch of your foot
(but stop short); keep your knee bent out to the
side. Repeat this action with your opposite leg.
(See fig. 11.2.)

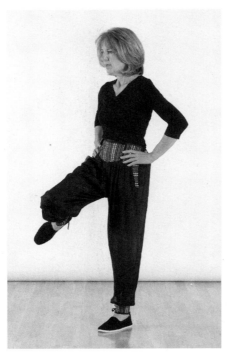

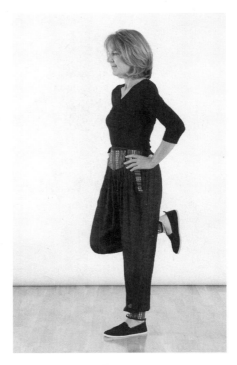

[11.3] [11.4]

Dog Kick

Lift your right knee and foot simultaneously, kicking out to the side like a urinating dog. Repeat on left side. (See fig. 11.3.)

Back Kick

Lift and flex your right foot to kick behind you toward your buttocks; make sure that your thigh stays straight (vertical to the ground) so you are only moving from the knee. Repeat this action on the left. (This can actually be a self-defense kick into the scrotum if a man comes up to you from behind. See fig. 11.4.)

Do each kick once in each direction. Complete four to eight rounds.

Twisting Crane

This crane movement helps strengthen the bladder muscles to prevent or cure incontinence and lift prolapsed pelvic organs.

1. Cross your right leg comfortably over to the outside of the left foot, with your right knee covering the left knee.

2. Bend your arms in an oval in front of your chest with your palms facing down and the middle fingers nearly touching. (See fig. 11.5.)
Inhale

3. Bend down so your knees fold in behind one another.
Exhale

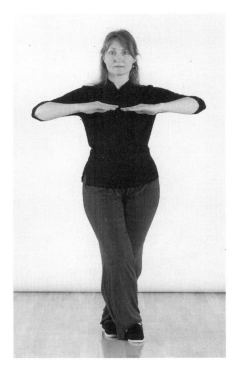

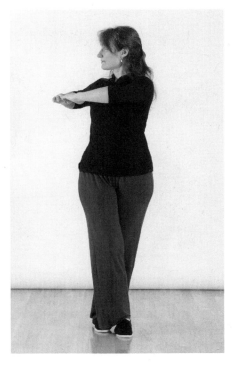

[11.5]   [11.6]

4. Twist to the right from your waist, and simultaneously straighten your legs and contract your lower abdominal muscles. (See fig. 11.6.)

5. Pull up on your pelvic floor and squeeze your thighs together. Focus on directing your energy upward into the bladder area in your lower abdomen. This squeezing movement stimulates the urinary sphincter, which often becomes flaccid with age. The main purpose is to pull the energy upward to counteract the downward force of a weak bladder.

Inhale

6. Rotate back to center, and bend your knees as before.

Exhale

7. Repeat the twist to the right and pull up on the pelvic floor.

Do this routine nine times to the right. Then switch your legs so the left foot crosses over to the outside of the right foot. Repeat the same twisting motions nine times to the left.

Crane Walk

The Crane Walk helps to strengthen the heart, calm emotions, and ease anxiety.

1. Begin in Basic Qigong Stance.
Inhale

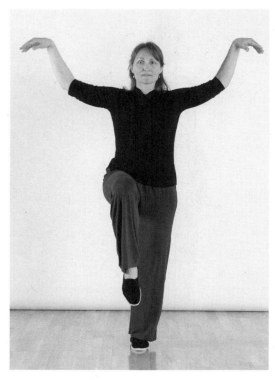

[11.7]

2. Lift your right leg so your thigh is parallel to the ground and point your toes.

3. Simultaneously raise your arms upward, imagining they are wings. Your arms will create a "U" as you bend your wrists and drape your fingers toward the ground. (See fig. 11.7.)

Exhale

4. Step down with your right foot, land on the heel, and rock forward as you take a step.

5. At the same time, lower your arms back to your sides like you're flapping your wings.

6. Then, raise your left thigh while lifting your arms up in the air again. The arm and leg lifts should be coordinated movements.

7. Continue walking slowly for one to three minutes, expanding your wings gracefully with each stride. On the exhalation you can quietly blow out through your mouth and say "haaa" as you walk.

This is a very relaxing walk that can be done anytime during the day—especially when you need to de-stress.

Nourishing the Uterine Palace

Breathing into the Uterine Palace nourishes the reproductive system and helps to moisten and preserve the epithelial lining of the vagina, which shrinks and becomes dry with age.

The Uterine Palace (see chapter 4, Activating Your Energy, p. 22 for more details) is found by placing your palms on the lower abdomen, with your thumbs on your belly button and index fingers forming the apex of a triangle with fingers pointing down toward your pubis. The point underneath the index fingers is the Uterine Palace.

1. Stand in Modified Horse Stance (legs bent about 2 to 3 feet apart). Place your index fingers on your Uterine Palace. Take a deep inhalation.

Exhale as you squat down.

Inhale

2. Slowly rise up, gently pulling up on the perineum, anus, and vagina.

3. Focus on drawing energy up to the Uterine Palace with each inhalation, invigorating your reproductive organs with fresh Qi.

4. You should feel your lower abdominal muscles gently expanding under your fingers.

Continue squatting and gathering the energy up into your Uterine Palace for twenty-four repetitions.

Dragon Spiraling up the Pillar

This movement stimulates the cerebral spinal fluid that bathes the spine and brain, maintaining flexibility in both body and mind. The twisting action will keep your back supple at the same time as it massages your internal organs. (Turn to chapter 17, Insomnia, p. 122 for a detailed description.)

Backward Walk or Run

The backward walk or run lays down new tracks in the brain by doing something totally different from your regular routine. It increases your mental acuity, improves coordination, and balances the hemispheres of the brain. Begin by walking or jogging slowly for ten to twenty steps and work up to one hundred or more. Make sure the path is level, without any obstructions, or you may fall flat on your butt! I find running backward to be very invigorating, and it clears my mind for a more productive day.

STANCES

Practice the Three-Circles Stance (see chapter 5, Stances, p. 31). Squat into a Modified Horse Stance (legs 2 to 3 feet apart) with your arms forming a circle out in front and your hands holding an invisible ball at eye level. Concentrate on slow *dantian* breathing. Begin slowly, standing for one to three minutes at a time; then gradually increase to ten minutes.

SELF-HEALING MASSAGE

Kidney Massage

Massage your kidney area below your ribs on your back. Rub with a loose fist or palm until the area is warm. It's important to keep the kidneys warm to invigorate the yang energy to maintain your vitality.

MEDITATION

Five-Eight Meditation

Inhale to a count of five, and exhale to the count of eight. The prolonged exhalation stimulates the parasympathetic nervous system, soothing and healing the body and relaxing the sympathetic fight-or-flight response. Begin sitting for three to five minutes; slowly build up to ten to fifteen minutes.

CONCLUSION

The Wise Woman Qigong will strengthen your bones, keep you flexible, and increase your coordination and balance. There are a myriad of symptoms that may arise during menopause or postmenopause, so augment your routine by adding exercises from the other chapters to address your imbalances. It's also important to practice the breast cancer prevention exercises twice a week or daily if breast cancer runs in your family (see chapter 14, Breast Health, p. 99).

This is a time in a woman's life that calls for her to honor herself and become attuned to her inner wisdom. Spend more time in solitude and allow your body to speak to you of its needs. Incorporate a spiritual component into your mind-body practice to deepen your gratitude for the wondrous gift of life.

12

Sage Woman

SIXTY-FIVE AND BEYOND

WHILE VISITING CHINA, I was impressed by the Chinese people's dedication to exercise. They met in the parks daily to stretch, dance, practice tai chi or Qigong, and socialize. I saw elders hanging out and sipping tea while draping a leg over a fence. One morning, as I was stretching after the long transoceanic flight, an old woman came over and swung her leg straight up to her ear, grinning widely at this bedraggled American. I was humbled.

In many countries where physical labor and outdoor activity are the norm, osteoporosis, obesity, and many of our common degenerative diseases are not prevalent. Women continue their daily routines well into their sage years. In China, diet also plays a strong role in supporting longevity—vegetables are their main source of nourishment, with very low ingestion of sugary foods. The emphasis they place on physical well-being, coupled with the historical respect they have for long life, has led to the subsequent development of mind-body disciplines that are an integral part of their cultural consciousness.

In my practice I have found that there is a wide variance in women's health concerns during these elder years, so I've designed an overall workout that most women can do without difficulty or strain. Use this as a template and include additional Qigong exercises that best meet your body's needs, such as those described in the Heart Health chapter if you have high blood pressure or cardiac concerns. Remember: this is *your* fitness program, so create a routine that resonates with your body and enables you to feel energized, strong, and balanced in mind, body, and soul.

DYNAMIC EXERCISES

Shoulder Shrugging and One-Foot Thud

Shoulder Shrugging is one of the most important movements to help prevent osteoporosis and rebuild bone. (See chapter 4, Activating Your Energy, p. 24.) The jarring of the bones sends a message to the brain that more calcium is needed and thus stimulates bone strength and rebuilding. Substitute the One-Foot Thud for the Shoulder Shrugging exercise if you find Shoulder Shrugging too strenuous or uncomfortable on your feet.

ONE-FOOT THUD

1. Place your feet hip-width apart and align the heel of your right foot with the middle of your left instep; place your right hand on the kidney area of your back.

Inhale

2. Keep your weight on your right leg as you lift up onto the toes of your left foot.

3. Swing your left arm upward and overhead as you raise up on your toes. (See fig. 12.1.)

Exhale

4. As you drop your left heel to the ground with a thud, let your arm fall back down to your side—both movements should occur simultaneously.

Continue this action thirty-six times. Switch sides and repeat. If you have osteoporosis or are in a weakened state, perform nine to eighteen times.

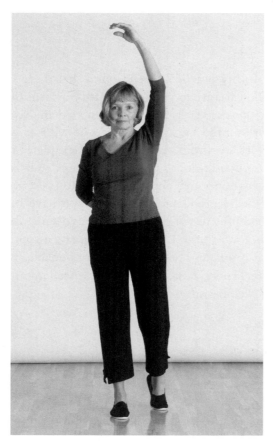

[12.1]

Side Hop

The Side Hop develops balance, coordination, and aerobic stamina, as well as improves your reflexes so you will be less likely to fall and injure yourself if you trip or if someone bumps into you.

1. Stand in Basic Qigong Stance. Hop sideways to the right on your right foot, with your left leg following so your feet come together.

2. As you hop, raise your right arm up to the side as if balancing against a wall, cross your left arm in front of your chest with your palm facing inward.

3. Then jump to the left and lift your left arm upward. Widen your stride as you get more comfortable with the movement. (See fig. 12.2.)

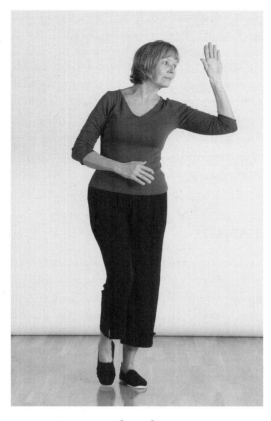

[12.2]

Complete twelve hops to each side, or if you're in good shape you can continue for two minutes. There is no particular breathing with the Side Hop, so do what feels natural to you.

Figure Eight Walk

This exercise moves Qi, regulates blood pressure, softens blood vessels, and improves coordination and overall balance. This is particu-

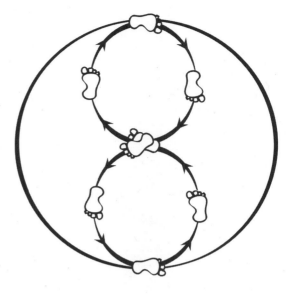

[12.3]

larly beneficial if you've had a stroke or heart problems.

1. Begin by drawing a large figure eight in the dirt—expansive enough so it will easily accommodate four natural steps from the center out to each side.

2. Mark your center point so it's visible.

3. Walk around one circle in four steps, coming back to the center, and trace four steps for the other circle. Try to keep the circles round and even. (See fig. 12.3.)

4. Bend your knees and swing your arms as you glide around the figure eight as though you are skating.

5. Your arms will move up and down depending on which side of the circle you are turning. For instance your left arm will be down as

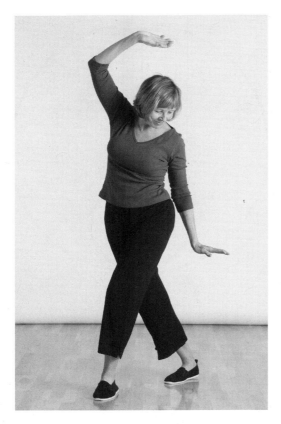

[12.4]

Heart's Gentle Rock and Simple Snake Movements

The Heart's Gentle Rock (see chapter 19, Heart Health, p. 137) will increase your circulation and benefit cardiovascular health by regulating your heart rhythm. The Simple Snake Movements will help you to regain elasticity in your upper body and to remain limber (see chapter 4, Activating Your Energy, p. 25).

STANCE

Stand in the Three-Circles Stance to develop your stamina and boost immunity. Focus on your *dantian* breathing while holding this pose. Begin by standing for one minute and gradually increase the duration of your stance to five minutes. (For a full description turn to chapter 5, Stances, p. 31.)

SELF-HEALING MASSAGE
Spiral Massage

Spiral Massage will stimulate digestion, help increase your appetite if it is low, and regulate the intestines.

your left side is inside the circle, with your right arm raised; then, as you cross over so your right side is inside the circle, your right arm will be down and your left arm will be overhead. (See fig. 12.4.)

Complete this eight times, then go back to your center point and begin another cycle commencing in the opposite direction; if you began walking to the right first, now you'll go to the left.

1. Stand in Basic Qigong Stance or lie down. Place your right hand on your belly button and rest your left hand atop your right.
2. Begin your massage by spiraling out in small clockwise circles and gradually increasing the circles to encompass the whole belly.

3. After twenty-four rotations, reverse the direction and massage another thirty-six times, slowly decreasing the size of the rotations as you circle inward back toward the center.

This is performed with the abdomen relaxed and the anus loose. You can do this in bed upon awaking and again before retiring at night.

MEDITATION

Five-Eight Meditation

This meditation will help regulate your nervous system and aid in relaxation, pain management, and sleep. Begin with a few minutes a day and gradually increase to ten to twenty minutes. (See full description in chapter 6, Meditation, p. 35.)

CONCLUSION

My teacher is the best example of someone who has kept fit solely by practicing Qigong. He has defined muscles, strength, balance, and abundant energy, yet doesn't do aerobics, weight lifting, yoga, or Pilates. He looks twenty years younger than his actual age! But Qigong isn't only successful with those who've practiced it for a lifetime. I've also seen bedridden patients and seniors who have never exercised be brought back to health by practicing Qigong.

Listen to your body, and at the very least do ten minutes of walking (such as *Guo Lin* Walking described in chapter 18, Breast Cancer, p. 130) or some other form of Qigong daily. The more you do, the fitter you'll become. You can live a long and productive life: visualize how you want to feel and move, and go for it! You're never too old to start Qigong.

PART THREE

Self-Healing for Women

13

Premenstrual Syndrome (PMS)

Eternally, woman spills herself away in driblets
to the thirsty, seldom being allowed the time, the quiet,
the peace, to let the pitcher fill up to the brim.

— ANNE MORROW LINDBERGH

PMS IS NO MYSTERY to most women. Many of us live on an emotional roller coaster with our hormones at the helm. We feel productive and ready to take on the world one week and the next week on the verge of tears at the slightest cross word. It wasn't until the 1980s that this affliction was taken seriously, since most Western doctors considered it purely psychosomatic.

In my practice I've come to understand PMS as a multifaceted disharmony. Stress plays a major role, along with poor diet, lack of exercise, and hormonal imbalances. In Chinese medicine the myriad symptoms of PMS typically involve the liver and spleen meridians, although all of the systems associated with reproduction can be affected. A harmonious menstrual cycle depends on the delicate interplay of the Qi, blood, emotions, and a woman's lifestyle choices. When balance in the body, mind, and spirit isn't maintained, then various PMS symptoms will occur throughout the monthly hormonal fluctuations.

The most common Chinese diagnosis for PMS is stagnant liver Qi, a prevalent condition in our society caused from overdoing, caffeine, and stress. At ovulation the liver energy is dominant, storing the blood to nourish the egg and then releasing the blood for menstruation. It controls the circulation of Qi throughout the body and is considered the temperamental organ, susceptible to emotional upset, anger, and suppressed feelings. Disrupted liver Qi will present the classical symptoms of PMS, such as frustration, anger, depression, headache, breast tenderness, and digestive problems. The other important meridian in PMS is the spleen, which oversees the production and control of blood, along with digestion. Resulting imbalances may manifest as abdominal bloating, sugar cravings, and digestive distress.

A deeper root cause of PMS, beyond the meridian imbalances, stems from our disconnection to our natural body rhythms. Women are intimately connected to the cycles of the moon. Our bodies experience the ebb and flow of our inner tides: emotions, hormones, and energies all wax and wane each month. Our busy lifestyles have made it inconvenient to notice these shifts, resulting in a continual struggle to keep up, no matter how we feel. If we begin to honor these changes, we'll naturally fall into more harmonious rhythms and connect intimately with our body's needs. Therefore, the most important focus in PMS treatment is to seek balance by incorporating a routine of self-care, such as Qigong and exercise, which can alleviate many common and nagging symptoms and regulate the menstrual cycle naturally.

I've treated many women with PMS with Oriental medicine, but teaching women how to redirect their emotional energies through Qigong has been the most successful therapy to sustain their monthly equilibrium. One of my patients, Lida, rushed into my office like a whirlwind, begging me to fix her tiny "bloated" stomach and then ran over to the mirror to check her eyes. "I can't go to work looking like this. I can't stand this puffiness. Please help me!" she cried. As a fashion designer, her looks were very important to her—both personally and professionally. Lida also had a history of anorexia and watched herself obsessively in the mirror for any signs of weight gain. The two weeks from ovulation to menstruation were a nightmare for her; she suffered with breast tenderness, abdominal bloating, and bouts of anger and anxiety. She also confided that she was in an abusive marriage but she was too afraid to leave and thus felt "stuck" in her life. She dealt with this by working overtime so she wouldn't have to face her unhappiness.

The underlying causes of Lida's PMS were her unexpressed emotions and inability to relax. Lida was the perfect candidate for the liver Qigong exercises to release her suppressed anger and reestablish a more harmonious flow to her life. I also included movements to nourish her Earth element (spleen and stomach), which had suffered from years of anorexia.

Since lifestyle modifications are essential in treating PMS (as well as most imbalances), we reviewed her diet and eliminated caffeine. This gave her immediate relief from breast distention, along with taking vitamin E (800 IUs) and evening primrose oil (500 milligrams) daily—the two supplements I recommend for cystic breasts. Following the recommended Qigong program (described later), she felt instant relief. She was able to handle her stress more effectively and she felt more even-keeled both emotionally and physically. Lida particularly enjoyed Push the Mountain, which released the anger she felt toward her husband. She also practiced Qigong breathing throughout her workday to ease anxiety. Eventually, her more balanced attitude enabled her to make big changes in her life, including seeking a divorce.

The treatment objective for PMS is to strengthen the spleen, move liver Qi stagnation, and calm the emotions. A commitment to daily Qigong (even if it's only for fifteen minutes) as well as walking (or another aerobic exercise) three to five times a week, will move the energy and keep it flowing. You'll notice a difference in how you feel immediately and most of your symptoms will be alleviated within one to two menstrual cycles.

DYNAMIC EXERCISES AND HEALING SOUNDS

Push the Mountain

This energetic exercise moves stagnant liver Qi and is the most effective emotional release exercise for PMS.

Push the Mountain

Push the Mountain will give you more vitality and stabilize emotions, especially anger and depression.

1. Move into the Horse Stance.
Inhale
2. Bend your elbows so they're approximately at a 90 degree angle and place your arms by your midtorso next to your ribs (adjacent to the liver and spleen).

3. Close your hands into a fist, with clenched fingers facing upward. (See fig. 13.1.)
Exhale
4. Rotate your forearms and open your hands so your palms face outward from the front of your body. Actively press your palms out as if pressing a wall away from you. At the end of the exhalation, your arms should be extended in front of your body at chest level. (See fig. 13.2.)
Inhale

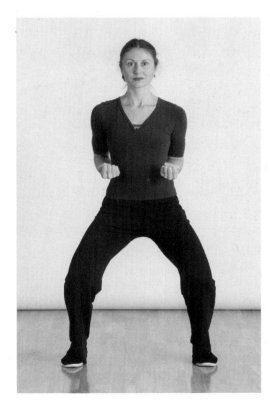

[13.1]

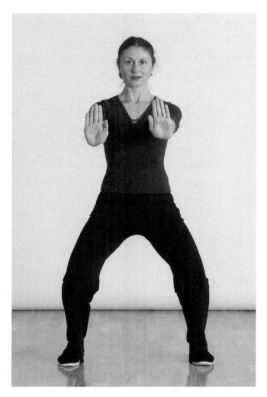

[13.2]

5. Pull your arms back and bring your fists back to your sides, so that they are in the starting position—your hands once again facing upward.

Release your anger, depression, and unwanted emotions out of your body as you exhale. This is a yang exercise and is very cleansing and energizing. Once you've completed this routine nine to eighteen times, place your hands on your *dantian* (a couple of inches below your belly button) and gather the energy back to your center with a few calming breaths.

Liver and Spleen Healing Sounds

These organ sounds will release your emotional blockages. Focus on letting go of anger, depression, and worry, which adversely affect the liver and spleen meridians. Imagine light streaming into your body and connect with the healing universal energies all around you. (For a full description of these exercises turn to chapter 8, Six Healing Sounds, pp. 53, 57.)

Soothing the Middle

Soothing the Middle is both a massage and an exercise to regulate the balance of Qi between the spleen, liver, and gallbladder meridians and helps to allay symptoms of digestive distress. Disharmonies in these meridians manifests as abdominal bloating, nausea, diarrhea or constipation, breast tenderness, cramps, moodiness, and fatigue.

1. Lie on your back. Place your palms flat on your inguinal grooves (the creases where your thighs join your torso) with your fingers pointing toward your feet. Space your hands approximately one inch apart on either side of your midline.
Inhale
2. Flex your feet so your toes are pointed toward your head. Slightly bend your knees, allowing your legs to drop open, splaying outward to stretch your inner leg muscles. Flexing your feet while turning them outward stimulates the liver and spleen meridians.
3. Press the heels of your hands against your

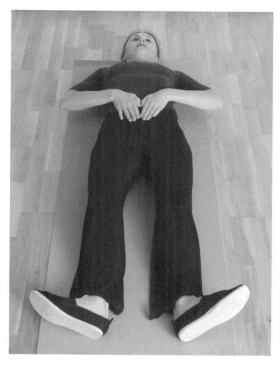

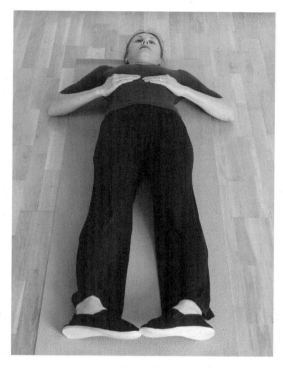

[13.3]

[13.4]

torso while slowly raising them to your ribs; keep your palms flat against your abdomen. (See fig. 13.3.)

Exhale

4. Draw your knees closer together as you stretch your feet into an inverted position (pigeon-toed) pointing your toes until the big toes touch. This stimulates your stomach meridian along your shins.

5. Move your palms sideways under your breasts, pressing your ribcage firmly. (See fig. 13.4.) Point your fingers downward, and continue to press as you extend your arms along the sides of your body toward your legs.

6. After exhaling completely, return your hands to starting position, resting them at the creases of your thighs and torso.

7. Move your hands to create two circles over your torso beginning at your pelvis, moving up to your sternum, across your ribs, and down your sides to the outside edge of your thighs, and then return to the inguinal grooves.

Combine the hand and leg movements into a synchronized flow. Perform a set of eighteen sequences morning and night. It is also possible to do this massage while standing, using only the hand movements. Focus on deep abdominal breathing and imagine the energy moving in your torso, soothing your internal organs.

STANCE

Awkward Stance

This stance will build your strength and increase the energy in your pelvis and reproductive organs. It's the best stance for healing gynecological problems; however, if it's too strenuous, then practice Three-Circles Stance to build your energy reserves. Maintain the posture for three minutes and gradually increase to ten minutes for optimal effects (turn to chapter 5, Stances, p. 31).

SELF-HEALING MASSAGE

Ren Mai *Massage*

Ren mai (also called conception vessel) is an acupuncture meridian that nourishes and regulates the reproductive system (see *Ren Chong* Meditation in chapter 6, Meditations p. 37, fig. 6.2). It extends up the front midline of the body and is responsible for the Qi flow in the abdomen as well as the chest and throat, areas that are also influenced by the liver meridian and prone to stagnation in PMS.

Inhale

1. Place your three middle fingers flat against your abdomen below the xiphoid process, the area below the breasts in the middle of your upper abdomen, just below the upward curve of your ribs. Never use firm pressure on this spot as it is a sensitive and fragile area.

Exhale

2. Massage downward along the midline from the xiphoid to the pubic bone with moderate pressure. Repeat this massage eighteen times.

MEDITATION

Ren Chong *Meditation*

Sit and gather your energy into these two important reproductive meridians for ten minutes after your Qigong practice (for a full description turn to chapter 6, Meditations, p. 36).

ADDITIONAL HEALING AIDS AND CONTEMPLATIONS

Herbs

The most popular Chinese herbal formula for PMS is Xiao Yao Wan, which can be prescribed for you by an acupuncturist or Chinese herbal practitioner. With stagnant liver Qi, this formula will diminish PMS in one to two cycles. Many people go to herbal pharmacies in Chinatown, where the herbal formulas are often not the highest quality (some are, for example, high in heavy metals), so it's best to buy from an acupuncturist whom you trust.

Diet

Avoid foods that are stimulating and spicy, especially right before your menses, because these will aggravate your liver. If you tend toward cramps, try taking calcium supplements (800 milligrams per day) ten days before you bleed to nourish your muscles and calm the nervous system.

The Emotional "Moon" Cycle

From the end of menstruation until ovulation is a time of expansive creative energy, corresponding to the ripening of the egg as the potential of life grows within us. This is a time when we tend to be more positive and productive, when possibilities and dreams abound. This blossoming peaks in ovulation, when the outward momentum then shifts toward receptivity, opening to impregnation in all aspects of our lives.

From ovulation to the menses, our focus goes inward and our intuitive abilities heighten. Many women become more sensitive to external stimuli, and if we're imbalanced, our underlying emotions are often ready to erupt, especially during the week prior to bleeding. This is when you want to divorce your husband for not cooking dinner when he promised, or lock the screaming kids in their rooms so you can nurse your headache in peace.

Menstruation is a time of cleansing and increased inner reflection. The best remedy is to spend some quiet time alone and nurture yourself. You can even train your family to expect this each month. Many women tell me they feel selfish when they do an activity just for themselves, without including the family. I remind them that they're not a bottomless well and they need to replenish so they can give to others from a place of fullness, self-respect, and love.

Contemplations to Deepen Your Healing

- Where do you feel stuck in your life and how can you change?
- How do you nourish yourself; what do you do just for you?
- How can you bring more balance into your life? What or who drains your energy and where do you need to say no?
- How do you express anger? Do you hold it in your body and where do you feel it settling?
- What are your natural rhythms within the lunar/menstrual cycle and how can you align your schedule to honor the flow of energy?

CONCLUSION

The deepest healing emerges when we acknowledge our emotional-physical rhythms and make the necessary lifestyle changes to achieve balance. Through Qigong practice, you learn to honor the feminine cycles as they continually shift in the dance of ripening, creating, and letting go each month. By cultivating a deeper sense of peace and acceptance of your body, you will become intimate with and responsive to your inner tides. With this new routine of Qigong self-healing, PMS can be reduced and even eliminated in a few cycles.

14

Breast Health

If the only prayer you ever say in your entire life
is "thank you," it will be enough.

—Meister Eckhart

Our breasts are vessels for nurturance, femininity, and sexuality, to be honored and cared for throughout our life. It's important to foster a positive attitude about your breasts regardless of the ideal image of the feminine physique that has been promoted through advertising in our country. We can't go anywhere without seeing Hollywood and recording stars revealing their perfectly round, voluptuous, and perky breasts. We're consumed by these projections from the moment our breasts emerge on our chests, worried that they're lopsided, too small to attract a mate, or too darn big to jog comfortably. They never seem to be "just right."

In ancient Chinese Taoist texts, the "milk chambers" were considered the center for spiritual cultivation for women. Adepts would concentrate Qi into their breasts through medi-

tation and Qigong, and then move this pure essence down to nourish their lower *dantian,* kidneys, and uterus. The breasts are connected to the uterus via the *chong* meridian, and so practicing breast Qigong will also indirectly benefit your uterus. The exercises described in this chapter will require you to breathe into your middle *dantian* (in the middle of your chest) to cultivate Qi in your chest and breasts (unlike other chapters where the exercises have you focus the energy below the belly button into your lower *dantian* or the Uterine Palace).

To maintain healthy breasts there are three important points to consider:

1. *Regulate Your Emotions.* Express your feelings and don't swallow them, especially anger (liver Qi), which has a deleterious effect on breast tissue. Try to solve your problems by

seeking to understand the situation from a positive perspective. In other words ask yourself: "What can I learn about myself from this circumstance?" rather than focusing on negative emotions. Since the stomach meridian also passes through the center of the nipple, is there a situation that you don't want to "stomach" anymore or where you need to speak your true feelings? Explore how you can nurture yourself with a mothering embrace.

2. *Diet as the Source of Nutrition.* What you choose to eat and how you nourish your body is extremely important. Avoid caffeine and fatty foods that tend to cause cystic lumps in breast tissue. Try to drink clean water and eat organic foods as much as possible, especially if you eat meat. Enjoy a wide palette of brightly colored foods, which are alive and full of Qi.

3. *Move! Move! Move!* Qigong and exercise prevent cancer and move liver Qi. Stagnant liver Qi is often responsible for cystic breasts and is especially common before the onset of menstruation. Get up and dance, walk, bike, or anything aerobic to keep your energy flowing and harmonized.

Although there is no guarantee that a woman won't contract cancer, it's imperative to be responsible for your own health as best you can. Many unhealthy breast conditions result from various degrees of stagnation of the Qi, blood, and fluids in the breasts, involving primarily the stomach, liver, and *chong* meridians. Unlike Western medicine, the Chinese see breast disease in a progressive pattern and can often trace the process from simple breast distension to tumors. Although there are different causes of stagnation contributing to breast lumps and tumors, this Qigong program will help maintain healthy breasts and the surrounding lymphatic tissue for overall breast health and cancer prevention.

DYNAMIC EXERCISES AND HEALING SOUNDS

This series of exercises and massages stimulates breast circulation and Qi flow in the lymph glands, particularly under the armpits and lateral sides of the breasts. This area becomes stagnant in our society since many women hold their arms pressed against their sides or across their chests or wear constricting bras. So relax your arms, take off that bra at home, and allow your breasts to breathe!

Breast Qigong should be integrated into your routine three times a week, given that there is an increase of breast cancer in women across America. You may want to perform this program daily if breast cancer runs in your family. Whenever you practice these exercises, it is important to send happy feelings to your breasts. Have a gentle smile on your face and appreciate your breasts with love and tenderness as you go through these movements. My teacher used to say to me: "Deborah, think, 'I am woman; I am beautiful; I am happy; I am healthy.'" Send joyous, nurturing Qi to your breasts.

Note: concentrate your breathing into the middle *dantian* (the energy center between the nipples in the center of your chest). Focus your attention on this area as you perform the Lymph Pump and all of the breast massages.

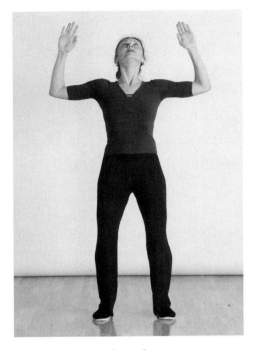

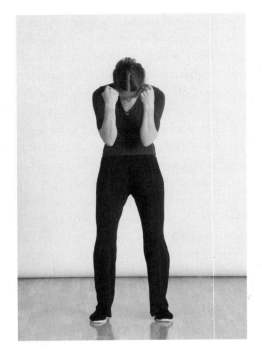

[14.1]   [14.2]

Lymph Pump

1. Stand in Basic Qigong Stance.

Inhale

2. Open your arms out to your sides with your elbows bent at 90 degrees, holding your forearms at shoulder level or above. Open your chest with a slight arch as you look upward. (See fig. 14.1.)

Exhale

3. Close your hands into fists and contract your arms into your chest as though you were performing a stomach crunch—pull your elbows against your torso. Look down. (See fig. 14.2.)

Repeat the Lymph Pump for a minute or longer. This action pumps the lymph system, which drains toxins from the blood and stimulates Qi flow in the chest. I do this invigorating exercise throughout the day to keep my energy flowing and expanded. You can breathe solely through your nose, or inhale through your nostrils and exhale through your mouth to increase detoxification.

THESE THREE ADDITIONAL Qigong exercises are also helpful for maintaining healthy breasts:

Liver Healing Sound

For a detailed description, refer to chapter 8, Six Healing Sounds, p. 53. Stagnant liver Qi is often tied to emotions such as depression, frustration, and anger, and can cause lumps and cystic breasts, so it's important to keep the Qi moving smoothly throughout the body with Qigong.

Spleen Healing Sound

For this exercise, see chapter 8, p. 57. The stomach and spleen meridians pass through and around the breasts, so they're vital for breast health. As you do the Healing Sound for the Spleen (which also affects the stomach, its paired organ), exhale worry and allow contentment and nurturance to bathe your chest.

Happy Liver Stretch

The Happy Liver Stretch soothes the emotions and opens the chest and underarm area, infusing your breasts with fresh Qi.

1. Stand in the Basic Qigong Stance with arms hanging at your sides.

Inhale

2. Place your left hand behind your lower back to support your spine as you arch slightly backward with this movement. Circle your right arm out in front and up overhead, stretching your arm with palm facing forward. (See fig. 14.3.)

Exhale

3. Sigh as you continue circling your arm back behind your torso, and then move it toward your side, completing the circle.

Repeat with the opposite arm: support your

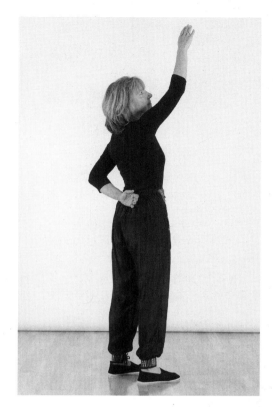

[14.3]

back with your right hand and circle your left arm. Continue for nine or eighteen times on each side or until you feel relaxed.

STANCES

Hugging the Tree Pose

By holding your arms in a circle at chest height, the Qi is stimulated in your breasts and arms to keep the Qi, blood and lymph moving. You may also project loving Qi to your breasts from the center of your palms and visualize healthy and beautiful breasts. For a full description turn to chapter 5, Stances, p. 30.

SELF-HEALING MASSAGE

If you've been diagnosed with breast cancer, *do not perform any* of the breast massages.

Nurturing Earth Yin Breast Massage

1. Stand in the Basic Qigong Stance. Begin by connecting with the Earth's energy and inhale her yin essence through the soles of your feet ("Bubbling Spring" is where Qi enters the body from the Earth). Then draw the Qi up the legs to your lower *dantian* (see chapter 10, Graceful Passage, figure 10.1, p. 71, for the point description and photo).

Inhale

3. Place your hands on your lower belly on either side of the midline. Press your palms flat against your body as you move them up your torso to your breasts. Continue to massage up the midline between your breasts.

Exhale

4. Circle your breasts with your palms going up and around the outer breast tissue; be sure to include the armpit and lymph area.

5. Continue circling your breasts with the palms of your hands: *inhaling* as you massage up the midline and *exhaling* as you press the outer breasts. (See fig. 14.4.)

6. After completing the eighth circle, slide your hands down the sides of your body to your thighs; imagine all of the toxins draining from your body and into the Earth to be transformed.

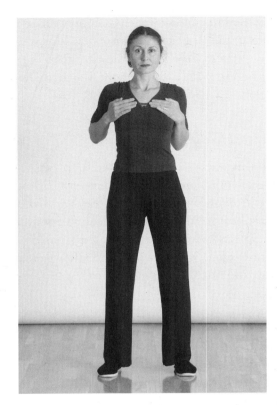

[14.4]

End the cycle by shaking out your hands for a moment.

7. Begin a new cycle, only this time it will be in the reverse direction. Start with your hands on your lower abdomen and pull your palms up your torso, then circle your breasts in the opposite direction eight times, going around to the outer edge of the breast first.

End by thanking the Earth for transmuting any toxins that you've released and take a moment to appreciate the nourishing yin energy that you've collected into your breasts.

Breast Snake Massage
(diagonal massage)

The snake technique is a Qigong massage utilized to gently move stagnation without hurting the tissue. This massage pumps the lymph in the breast and moves the Qi and blood.

Before massaging your breast, practice on your thigh to get the motion and pressure smooth.

1. Lay your palm flat against your thigh. Begin to undulate your palm by putting pressure first on the heel of your palm and then rolling up through the palm to your fingers, in a wave-like motion.

2. Gently lift the heel of your palm and resume pressing as you continue the wavelike movement with your fingers and hand, slowly inching forward.

Once you have the rhythm of this action, place your left hand behind your head with the elbow splayed outward as if you were to begin a self-exam. Massage your breast using a snake-like motion across the breast toward the armpit. Slowly press upward from the bottom of the breast along a diagonal line toward your armpit. For most breasts it takes three passes across them to cover all of the tissue and lymph areas. (See fig. 14.5.)

1. First, pass from the breastbone at the center of your chest (the lower medial corner of your breast) diagonally across to the armpit.

2. Next, start with your fingers below the breast and pass through the nipple and up to

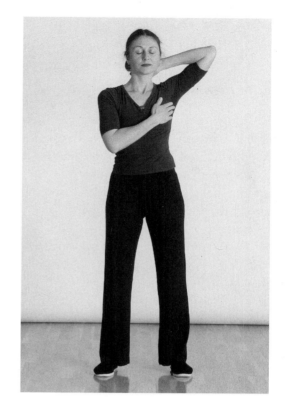

[14.5]

the armpit, massaging the lymph nodes in the underarm.

3. Last, pass along the outer edge of the breast tissue to the armpit.

If you have large breasts (or small hands) and don't cover the whole breast in these three passes, add more lines to be sure to cover all of the areas described. Each pass should be done three times. Then switch sides and do the other breast (i.e., the right breast with the right hand behind the head). This gentle snake massage increases circulation in the breast tissue and is particularly good for fibrocystic breasts or breasts with benign lumps.

Figure Eight Massage

1. Stand in Basic Qigong Stance. Take a moment to breathe in the Mother Earth energy through your feet; fill your whole body. Allow your breasts to receive this nurturing energy. Place one hand atop the other with palm flat against your lower belly.

Inhale

2. Move your hands up the midline to your breasts.

Exhale

3. Circle around one breast.

Inhale

4. Move your hands up the midline again.

Exhale

5. Circle around the other breast, creating a lateral figure eight or infinity symbol (∞) around your breasts.

Continue for eight rotations or more. Your hands should always go upward on the sternum (middle of the chest) with each inhalation, and around a breast on the exhalation. Do slow, rhythmic movements to stimulate the Qi, blood, and lymph circulation.

Nipple Rebound

After doing the breast massages, end with pressing your nipples with the palms of your hands three times. Press in and pull out quickly. This is called rebound pressure. This spring action helps clear the mammary ducts.

Breast Lift

This exercise tones the muscles around the breasts and helps prevent sagging. Clasp your wrists behind your back and flap your arms like wings, back and forth. You should feel your chest expanding to stimulate and move breast Qi. Continue for thirty-two to forty-eight flaps. This exercise moves the Qi and blood in the breasts as it lifts breast tissue and helps to shape the breasts (and keeps gravity from winning!).

MEDITATION
Ren Chong *Meditation*

Ren Chong Meditation moves the energy through the chest and abdomen and will complement the Breast Health routine by maintaining a harmonious flow of Qi and blood through these meridians and your breasts. For a full description see chapter 6, Meditation, p. 36.

ADDITIONAL HEALING AIDS AND ADVICE
Herbs and Supplements

If you suffer from cystic breasts, eliminate caffeine from your diet and take daily doses of vitamin E (400–800 IUs) and evening primrose oil (500 milligrams), an essential fatty acid containing gamma linoleic acid (GLA), which helps regulates sex hormones to alleviate mood swings, cramps, and breast tenderness. Both of these supplements are readily available in health food stores.

Castor Oil Packs

Applying castor oil packs helps reduce and often eliminate lumps such as cysts and fibroid adenomas often found in breast tissue.

Years ago I worked as an herbalist in an alternative health clinic. During this time I consulted with Sharon, a director of a metropolitan breast clinic, who was looking for a natural therapy to help alleviate the suffering many of her patients experienced due to lymphatic swelling and pain after mastectomies. I suggested they apply castor oil packs (an Edgar Cayce remedy) to their breasts.

She was skeptical when I first suggested this remedy, so she decided to experiment on herself at home first. She was delighted at how soothed and relaxed she felt during the process. When I saw her a year later, Sharon was still pleasantly surprised by the results she witnessed, especially with women who'd had mastectomies—sharing that it had become routine in the clinic. Sharon introduced this homespun remedy to hundreds of women in the hospital and was excited to report that the packs relieved lymphatic swelling and pain for all of the women; in fact, for many women, their lumps completely disappeared.

Many health food stores sell a cloth pack and castor oil treatment kit, or you can make your own by purchasing cotton flannel and castor oil from the drugstore. Since our skin is the largest organ of our body, I recommend using organic castor oil to reduce the amount of toxins absorbed into your body.

Place the cloth in a glass cooking dish and saturate it with castor oil. Warm it up in a microwave or in the oven. Next, get plastic wrap, a towel, and a hot water bottle (or a heating pad). Lie in your bed and place the oil-soaked flannel over your breasts, wrapping under your armpit if you have lymphatic congestion. If you want to secure the cloth, wrap your chest with the plastic wrap and then cover the pack with a towel. If you decide not to wrap yourself in plastic, be sure to spread a sheet of plastic underneath your body, with a towel on top to protect your linens. Castor oil is viscous like motor oil and will soil your clothes and sheets. Put a heat source on top of the castor oil pack and rest for an hour or so.

Although this may seem like a hassle, the whole process can be very comforting and healing, especially if you use this time to engage in a healing visualization. If this seems too time-consuming or messy, you can massage the heated oil into your breasts before bed. Wear an old shirt and lie on a spare towel. This is not a romantic adventure but it really works!

CONCLUSION

Many women confide that they are afraid to do self-exams for fear of finding a lump, but it's important to get acquainted with your own unique breast tissue and know if it has changed. Currently an astonishing number of women (one in eight), will get breast cancer in this country. Most breast cancers are initially found by women or their partners, so begin to perform your own checkup on a monthly basis.

Incorporating breast Qigong into your weekly routine is important to maintain shapely and healthy breasts and to prevent breast cancer. If you have breast cancer in your family, follow the routine daily or at least three times a week. You can also massage your breasts in the shower or while sitting in bed. Add these massages to your Qigong practice or create your own personal routine that will ensure that you honor and nurture your breasts.

15
Depression

This being human is a guest house. Every morning
a new arrival. A joy, a depression, a meanness, some
momentary awareness comes as an unexpected visitor.
Welcome and entertain them all! Even if they're a crowd
of sorrows, who violently sweep your house empty
of its furniture, still, treat each guest honorably.
He may be clearing you out for some new delight.

—RUMI

DEPRESSION HAS GROWN exponentially in our society, where the focus on material wealth and ego distraction has left our souls bereft. More people are beginning to question if there is a grander purpose to their lives and are seeking answers through meditation, spirituality, and religion. There are many forms of depression: situational depression related to grief and loss, seasonal affective disorder, as well as depression caused by chemical and hormonal imbalances or disharmonies of the organ systems. For the most part we will be discussing the more mild to moderate types of depression, often heralding a necessary journey into oneself to reveal deep emotions and unfulfilled desires. Qigong can help you attune to your inner landscape and explore some of the feelings that may emerge with depression.

Chinese doctors were among the first to acknowledge that the state of mind impacts a person's health. They observed that lingering emotions can hamper the organs and cause disease if not properly expressed. Both depression and anger are associated with a liver meridian imbalance: depression often occurs when anger is turned inward and repressed. This is especially prevalent in our culture, where women are conditioned to believe it's unladylike for them to express anger. Although this view might seem antiquated, the image is still embedded in our consciousness, especially within the older generations. The Chinese treatment principle is to "express it out"—whether it's anger, depression, or sadness. Don't rely on antidepressants, which further suppress your emotions and mask the core of your feelings.

If you go to an acupuncturist to be treated for depression, you'll probably be diagnosed with some degree of liver Qi stagnation since it's the most common causative factor of depression in this country. In addition to depression, you may also experience some of the other symptoms signaling stuck liver Qi: moodiness, irritability, roller-coaster emotions that worsen prior to menstruation, tension, headaches, breast distention, digestive problems, and menstrual irregularity. These symptoms are aggravated by stress, lack of exercise, hot and spicy foods, and stuffing your feelings. With depression, you want to keep moving and not get stifled by inactivity of your body or thoughts. Move (even though you may not feel like it) and you'll feel much better.

Some people who suffer from depression often have a lackluster appearance with an overall tenor of emptiness. This affects their heart energy, and women may also exhibit other symptoms, such tiredness and sullenness, paleness, difficulty falling asleep, anxiety, excessive crying or laughing (empty cheerfulness), dizziness, or heart palpitations. Whatever the cause of your depression, it's important to address it honestly and not let it linger. Studies reveal that people with untreated (or unresolved) depression are five times more likely to have a heart attack or heart problems, conditions that become more common as a woman ages.

In my clinic I've been able to wean many women off of antidepressants by alleviating stagnant liver Qi, nurturing their Heart (Fire) and Earth energies, and building and renewing their bodies and spirits. One of my most memorable patients was Annie, a charismatic woman in her midforties who was a successful Hollywood producer. She was a driven career woman, always on the go, working late into the night. She was the type of person who bolstered everyone around her, so I was surprised when she came to me desperate to get off Prozac and regain her emotional stability.

I prescribed a Qigong routine that focused on soothing her liver Qi, as well as a Saint-John's-wort tincture (see Additional Healing Aids). I told her we'd wean her off the Prozac in slow, incremental steps. In Annie's typical "let's do it now" fashion, she called me a week later and announced that she had quit the medication and was feeling like herself again! This is not how I usually like to work, but she was amazed at her new attitude and invigoration after a week on the herbal and Qigong routine. She remained off of antidepressants and referred her friends for the same program. I've also seen great success without herbal therapy, so try the Qigong first and see how you do for a month with consistent daily practice.

DYNAMIC EXERCISES AND HEALING SOUNDS

These exercises are beneficial for mild to moderate depression. If you suffer from prolonged, severe clinical depression or mental disorders, it's important for you to consult your health practitioner to receive proper medical treatment.

Warm-up

Practice the Whole-Body Pat (see chapter 4, Activating Your Energy on p. 24). This will help move stuck Qi and get the energy flowing throughout your body. It's energizing and can be done anytime during the day.

Body Shake

Stand comfortably and take a few big breaths. Begin to shake your limbs, and then let your whole body go and shake off any clinging energies, memories, and worries. Make sounds as you shimmy. Have you ever seen a child tremble when they're mad? They spontaneously release their anger and then return to playing moments later. Let it go!

Happy Liver Stretch

This simple exercise of alternate arm swings reduces stress by opening the Qi flow in the sides of the body and releasing stagnation both through stretching and sighing. For this exercise, see chapter 14, Breast Health, p. 101.

Snake

This movement is taken from the Shaolin Temple snake series that I do regularly to stimulate the flow of energy throughout my body and pelvis. It moves Qi, nourishes yin, and stimulates the sexual energy that is usually subdued by depression.

1. Stand in Basic Qigong Stance with your arms relaxed by your side. Slowly begin undulating your body back and forth (not side to side!) as if you were a snake. Begin the movement by pushing your sacrum/pelvis forward and then allow the wave to flow up through your torso and chest.
2. Scoop your lower body forward, initiating the movement that gently pushes your belly and chest forward and back in a long undulating wave. (See figs. 15.1 and 15.2.)
3. Feel this sensual motion within your body, rhythmic and smooth like a snake moving along its path.

Continue for one minute or longer. As you practice, the undulation will become subtler and you can experience the Qi initiating the wave from the Earth through your body or emerging through your vagina.

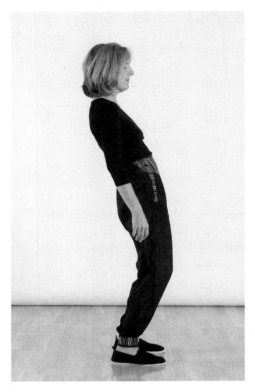

[15.1]

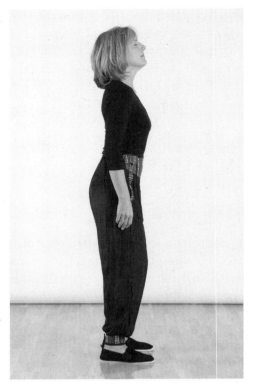

[15.2]

Push the Mountain

This exercise moves stagnant liver Qi and releases stuck emotions. It will activate your Qi and pull you out of the doldrums. (Turn to chapter 13, PMS, p. 93 for a full description.)

Six Healing Sounds

You can alternately practice the Liver (Wood), Heart (Fire), and Spleen (Earth) sounds, depending on your emotional needs of the day. Or you can do all of the Six Healing Sounds to regulate your entire body.

- Spleen: to dispel worry or if you're seeking more grounding
- Heart: when you're more anxious or sad
- Liver: if you're angry, grumpy, or feeling numb

These exercises are fully described in chapter 8, Six Healing Sounds.

STANCE

Practice the Awkward Stance: begin by holding it one to three minutes and build your endurance slowly. This posture stimulates the liver meridian and will allay stagnant energy to help heal depression. If you find it too difficult, then stand in Three-Circles Stance. (For full descriptions turn to chapter 5, Stances.)

SELF-HEALING MASSAGE

Liver 3 Massage

Run your finger along the groove between your first and second toes (first and second metatarsal bones bilaterally). There will be a tender acupuncture point, Liver 3, in a depression about an inch up from the big toe. I call this the

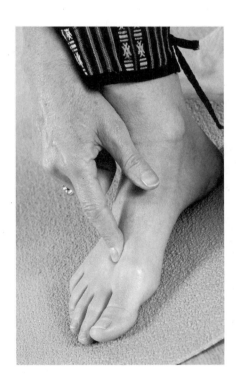

[15.3]

"stress point" since it harmonizes the emotions and spirit by regulating the movement of Qi throughout the mind-body. Massage this point as often as you want. (See fig. 15.3.)

MEDITATION

Floating Cloud Visualization

Lighten your mood with this visualization anytime you're feeling overwhelmed and heavy with depression or despair. Turn off the electronics, put aside any distractions, and set the mood for some nurturing time alone. Lie down or sit comfortably so you're very relaxed.

1. Take ten deep abdominal breaths and slowly sink into yourself.
2. Imagine that you're a cloud or riding atop a puff of clouds. Reflect on the qualities of clouds: light, buoyant, and changing.
3. Now feel these qualities within yourself. Sense the lightness of your body, the fleeting nature of your thoughts and emotions.

Simply rest and allow yourself to float aimlessly, like a cloud drifting by on a lazy summer's day. No cares, no worries. Float as long as you like!

Sea Meditation

This meditation will support you to move beneath the external stressors of your life and hopefully discover an underlying source of support and "rightness" of how your life is unfolding, despite external appearances. Do this for about ten to twenty minutes. (For a full description turn to chapter 6, Meditation, p. 35.)

ADDITIONAL HEALING AIDS AND CONTEMPLATIONS

Saint-John's-Wort

Fresh Saint-John's-wort tincture is one of my favorite herbal medicines that I've used successfully for over fifteen years. The small yellow blooms turn deep crimson when steeped in alcohol. Make sure that the tincture was made with fresh flowers, since the flowers lose potency when dried (the label should state this). This herbal remedy has been used in Europe for many years and is a standard prescription for depression. In the last ten years it has become popular and is now available in most health food stores. (I've found the tincture is more effective than capsules, if you're buying from a conventional drug or health food store in America.)

Singing and Dancing

Sing and chant. There's a Native American saying that if you're singing, you can't be depressed. It's true. Try it! Also dancing, even around the house, is great therapy.

Contemplations to Deepen Your Healing

- Are you really depressed or are you harboring resentments or anger that you've not released?
- What is your soul asking of you right now in your life?
- Are you depressed because you're not following your heart or intuitive guidance?
- Is your life purpose calling but you're afraid to step into the unknown?
- As Mary Oliver asked in her wonderful poem "The Summer Day": *"Tell me, what is it you plan to do with your one wild and precious life?"*[1]

CONCLUSION

"Melancholy gives the soul an opportunity to express a side of its nature that is as valid as any other, but is hidden out of our distaste for its darkness and bitterness. . . . For the soul, depression is an initiation, a rite of passage."[2]

— THOMAS MOORE

Depression as a journey into oneself may mark a necessary descent into what Thomas Moore and others have called the "dark night of the soul." This rite of passage is often considered negative, delving into those parts of ourselves that we'd rather ignore or hide in the basement. However, descending into our soul's depths is essential for self-awareness and inner growth. This journey is a vital part of an initiatory process spoken of by many spiritual traditions throughout the world. Each tradition describes a way to hold a piece of the light that will enable us to descend, but in the end we must find our own way home. I think of a lofty tree with branches spreading upward to the sky, yet hidden beneath are deep roots anchoring her into the Earth. This rootedness in our own life is what all of us must find for ourselves, and depression can be a call to begin this journey.

Qigong will help you access the depths of your feelings and release the stagnancy in your mind, emotions, and body. Movement unveils the cloak of despair, encouraging a balance between introspection and activity, so surrender to your feelings and express them freely as you follow your new Qigong program.

16

Menopause

I have enjoyed greatly the second blooming . . .
suddenly you find—at the age of fifty, say—
that a whole new life has opened before you.

— AGATHA CHRISTIE

MENOPAUSE IS NOT a disease but a rite of passage. The Chinese refer to menopause as the "second spring," a time to reflect, become acquainted with yourself, and contemplate life. In some indigenous cultures this passage of women moving into their wisdom years is the time to acknowledge them for all that they have contributed: raising the family, caring for the community, healing, or whatever their work has been. They are honored as elders, and some become the shamans or spiritual counselors for their community. Since this perspective is not inherent in our society, many women need to reframe menopause away from being a physical malady needing to be cured (or endured) to a time for them to come into their own power and uniqueness, often through renewed self-expression and creativity.

Menopause marks the cessation of menstruation and fertility, but it doesn't preclude us from being sexually attractive and dynamic throughout our lives, even as we age. My Qigong teacher often reminds me that aging is a wholesome process and that we should not look at menopause separately: birth, aging, and death are all part of the life cycle. When I complain about my wrinkles, he chides me, "Aging is a natural process—you can't reverse to a young girl," although Hollywood and cosmetic companies would like us to believe we can!

Many American women have the "it won't happen to me" syndrome, as if they're immune to aging. Then they come to my clinic for fatigue, mood swings, hot flashes, or insomnia and wonder what's going on. Some women have expressed that they don't recognize their bodies anymore, especially when looking down upon the emerging tummy roll. Menopause affects everyone differently. Some women have symptoms for years while others sail through without notice.

In my menopausal Qigong classes, the most comical and challenging issue is regulating the temperature in the room to suit everyone. In winter, some women shiver with the windows open while others are frantically fanning their dripping chests. Complaints fly around the group about hot flashes, insomnia, relationship tensions, depression, and lack of sexual desire. Many truly want a "pause from men," and Prozac is not the answer!

The kidney energy is responsible for reproduction and growth cycles. Young girls begin bleeding between the ages of eleven and fourteen, with major shifts occurring in seven-year increments. By the time women reach age forty-nine, a natural decline has been slowly taking place as the kidney yin and yang wane, blood production slows down, and digestion isn't as robust as before.

Since the emotion associated with the kidneys is fear, many old feelings and anxieties we thought were resolved will often resurface. Concerns of losing our attractiveness and declining sexual libido may emerge, and our self-image often wrinkles (literally) in front of our eyes. Part of this change is physiological, but a huge component is seated in our self-perception. What will happen to us as we lose our youthful appearance? Who are we without our children, husband, or mate? What is our purpose and how do we want to spend the rest of our lives?

The Chinese traditionally view change as part of the natural flow of life. From this spiritual perspective, it's advised to embrace transition in our lives as simply as we do the weather. Suffering comes from resistance, so it's helpful to understand and embrace our fears. As Dr. Wu says, "Everything changes. This is life. Accept and recover from your wounds. Cope with change or change with change."

Remember that you are the guardian of your own health. Western women tend to think of menopause as an ailment that needs to be corrected. They will often rush to the pharmacy or the doctor to get supplements or drugs to fix the "problem"—often causing more troubles in the process. The most common solution is to use estrogen or synthetic hormones to adjust the hormonal imbalance, yet this disrupts the natural cycles of your body. For example, at menarche breasts develop through natural estrogen stimulation, but if you push the cells with estrogen at menopause, it can cause a negative reaction, like cancer. As teenagers it's rare for girls to develop breast cancer, since the breasts have a natural affinity to estrogen that declines as we age. Qigong will give you the tools and the ability to go through this passage without the use of extra hormones and drugs.

Some of the common concerns I've treated in my clinic with Qigong are lowered libido, weight gain, joint stiffness/pain, hot flashes, insomnia, anxiety, memory loss, and fatigue. Menopausal symptoms can be alleviated with

Qigong exercises, meditation, and a sound diet. It is also helpful to be involved in a creative project or community activity, or to have group support during this time. Finding balance is key to a stress-free passage, allowing quiet, reflective moments alone as well as with friends.

You can mix the exercises from this chapter together with the ones for your age group to design your own Qigong routine. This is not like tai chi, where you need to follow one form. It is important that you enjoy your practice so you'll feel inspired and strengthened.

DYNAMIC EXERCISES AND HEALING SOUNDS

Sweeping Water

This movement nourishes the kidney energy. As you exhale, imagine releasing your fears and anxieties and replacing them with trust and faith. Remember, focusing your intention amplifies the effects of Qigong.

1. Stand with your feet about 3 feet apart, knees slightly bent. Curl your left hand into a loose fist and place it on your right kidney area (on your back, just above your waist).

2. Place your right forearm parallel to your chest and about a foot in front, with your forearm parallel to the ground, palm facing down.

Inhale

3. Slowly shift your weight to the right; you will be tracing a half circle with your right hand/arm.

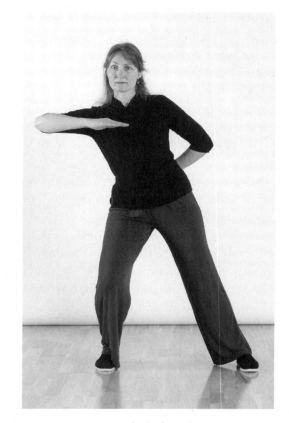

[16.1]

4. Keep your forearm parallel to the ground as you sweep your arm out to the right side—leading with the elbow. (See fig. 16.1.) Then open your arm out completely, moving your forearm until it's extended to your right side. Imagine you're skimming the top of a lake with your palm. At this point your arm should be parallel to the floor and about 90 degrees from your body.

Exhale

5. Slightly bend down as you continue sweeping your arm in a semicircle down and in

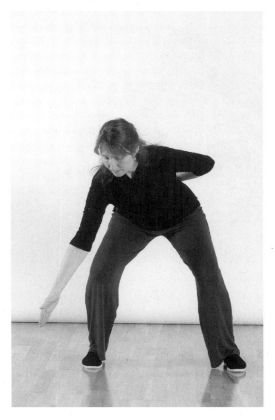

[16.2]

front of you and scoop your arm up to the left side. (See fig. 16.2.)

6. Shift your weight with the movement: first to the right, the center, and then over to the left.

Inhale

7. Come back to the starting position. Continue again to the right, circling nine times to the right, then change directions and circle with your left hand.

This movement is a slow, continuous sweep, like a waterwheel. Move gracefully and smoothly, like water.

Push the Mountain

This is usually the favorite menopausal exercise in my classes for releasing pent-up emotions, especially anger, and revitalizing the body. (For a full description turn to chapter 13, PMS, p. 93.) Be sure to perform this exercise prior to the Pelvic Tilt (chapter 21, Restoring Sexual Qi, p. 151) and Pelvic Floor Lift (described below). Do this movement nine to eighteen times.

Pelvic Floor Lift

The Pelvic Floor Lift increases Qi and blood flow in the pelvic floor, strengthens the lower back and hips, and helps heal incontinence.

1. Lie on your back with knees bent, feet on the floor, a little wider than shoulder-width apart. Bring your heels back toward your buttocks so you can touch your heels with your middle fingers as your arms lay relaxed by your sides.

Inhale

2. Breathe into the Uterine Palace for the entire inhalation and movements.

3. Open your knees so they fall out to the side, while keeping the outer edge of your feet on the floor.

4. Lift your hips upward and settle your weight on your upper back and shoulders.

5. Bring your knees closer together, as though you're squeezing your partner between your legs. Your knees should be about a foot

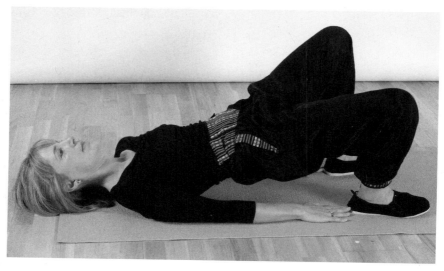

[16.3]

apart. (This is similar to the yoga Bridge Pose. See fig. 16.3.)

Exhale

6. Slowly lower your buttocks to the floor and begin the sequence again.

Repeat this exercise nine to eighteen times.

Triple Heater and Kidney Healing Sounds

The Triple Heater Healing Sound will help relieve insomnia, hot flashes, night sweats, agitation, and anxiety by regulating the temperature throughout your body, as well as relieving excess heat. The kidneys nourish the yin and essence of a woman and support the heart. (For a full description of these exercises turn to chapter 8, Six Healing Sounds, pp. 56 and 52 respectively.)

STANCE

Do the Awkward Stance to stimulate the yin meridians and nourish the spleen, liver, and kidney energies. This will strengthen your whole body, especially your legs, and increase immunity, vitality, and balance (with the added bonus of firming your butt and thighs!). If it's too difficult, then do the Three-Circles Stance. Begin with one to three minutes and slowly work up to ten to fifteen minutes if you can.

SELF-HEALING MASSAGE

Ovary Massage

This massage will help slow the decline of the hormones by stimulating the ovaries. Massaging will soothe the lower abdomen and reproductive organs and alleviate menopausal symptoms.

1. Stand in Basic Qigong Stance. Place both your thumbs in your belly button and form a triangle with your index fingers pointing downward. Your middle fingers will be over your ovaries.

2. Place your palms flat against your lower abdomen. (Refer to fig. 4.2, p. 22.)

3. Massage down and outward in circles, keeping your palms flat against your belly and your thumbs over your umbilicus.

Try to relax your shoulders and don't strain. Do this massage 60 to 180 times or until your belly is warm.

MEDITATION

It is very helpful to implement a meditation practice to navigate a smooth sail through menopause. I had a friend share that her insomnia was alleviated when she was at a meditation retreat, but as soon as she returned home, so did her restless sleep. Meditation settles the mind and spirit and is a yin activity, still and quiet, so I believe it will nourish your yin as well. Begin or end your day with ten to twenty minutes of Mindfulness Meditation (chapter 6, Meditations, p. 34), focusing your attention on the inhalation and expiration of your breath. The most important element is consistency; allow time and space to train the mind and dip into a deeper place of inner solace—essential for re-framing menopause as a time for reflection and transition.

After your Qigong workout, sit for ten minutes to direct energy into your *ren* and *chong* meridians as you perform the *Ren Chong* Meditation (chapter 6, Meditations, p. 36). This will help nourish your yin, fluids, and blood to help counter hot flashes, night sweats, and dryness.

If you find you're very emotional and sensitive, then practice the *Dunhuang* Meditation (chapter 6, Meditations, p. 36). This is a cleansing meditation that expels negativity, releases tension, and calms the mind. Stand or sit for five to ten minutes daily.

ADDITIONAL HEALING AIDS AND CONTEMPLATIONS

Herbs and Diet

There are many herbal formulas available to reduce or eliminate the symptoms of menopause. Have your acupuncturist prescribe an appropriate herbal remedy to meet your needs. Eat plenty of dark, leafy green vegetables and soy products, and moderate your sugar, caffeine, and alcohol consumption, all of which exacerbate hot flashes.

Contemplations to Deepen Your Healing

• Where do you need to take a "pause" in your life?
• Do you yearn for more reflective time alone?

- Is a creative project calling you?
- Do you have a spiritual practice that nurtures your soul?
- Is your work satisfying, or have you been considering a change to something that really impassions you?
- Where's the fire in your life right now, besides the hot flashes?

It might be beneficial for you to participate in a rite of passage for yourself with friends or alone as a way to mark the releasing of your youth and unrequited dreams, and to embrace your wise woman years of wisdom, creativity, and spirituality.

CONCLUSION

During menopause it's imperative to focus on mind-body regulation and become proactive in all levels of your well-being: emotional, physical, mental, and spiritual. Qigong harmonizes these synergistic relationships to help you achieve optimum health. By defining your inner and outer practices, you can age gracefully and ripen into your later years with dignity and vitality.

17

Insomnia

You ought not attempt to cure the body without the soul.
The cure of many diseases is unknown to many physicians
because they disregard the whole.

—HIPPOCRATES

INSOMNIA CAN MANIFEST in various ways: difficulty falling asleep, restless slumber, early morning waking (especially around 3:00 A.M.), and dream-disturbed sleep. The Chinese say that the mind needs to be "rooted" in a healthy heart or else it floats at night and has no place to rest. If there's deficiency of blood or yin or excess emotions affecting the heart, then the *Shen* (spirit) is restless. In fact, imbalances of any organ, as well as labile emotions, can disturb the mind and spirit.

Insomnia seems to appear during perimenopause and often stays for years if not addressed. Insomnia can be debilitating, dampening one's whole perspective on life and may even weaken the immune system since the body repairs itself at night. The encouraging news is that I've witnessed numerous women who practice Qigong exercises, coupled with the calming *dantian* breathing, cure their insomnia without medication—some as quickly as within a week and other, more chronic cases, in about three to six months.

A healthy liver is also important to sleep since it controls and stores the blood, which nourishes the heart and entire body. Many women wake between 1:00 and 3:00 A.M.—the time of the liver—indicating an imbalance in this meridian. There may be deficient blood (evident in many menstruating women) or deficient yin creating heat, often typical with menopausal women who experience night sweats stemming from a liver and/or kidney imbalance. The spleen, which produces the blood, can also be affected by overthinking and worry, a common habit when lying in bed trying to fall asleep. Any excessive emotional state can hinder sleep, so try to leave the thinking out of the bedroom!

It is important to create a space conducive to healthy rest. Buy an air filter if allergies keep you awake. Ensure a dark and quiet room with adequate ventilation and don't sleep next to an electric clock or computer as they can affect your electromagnetic field. Become more aware of your behavior in preparing for sleep. Cut out stimuli before bedtime like eating (requiring digestive energy), indulge in sweets or alcohol, or watching TV or action movies (including the news!). If you're sensitive to caffeine don't drink coffee and tea after the morning hours, especially during perimenopause/menopause when you may become more sensitive to stimulants.

Substitute relaxing preludes to sleep such as taking a luxurious bath with lavender oil, or listening to calming music, or meditating. Journal or discuss the day with your partner before bed. Save the planning until the next morning!

While sleep aids or medication may work well, they won't heal your insomnia. Although Qigong takes more time, it will eventually harmonize the mind-body imbalance. Coupled with self-massage and slow *dantian* breathing, this Qigong program will regulate your sleep naturally.

DYNAMIC EXERCISES AND HEALING SOUNDS

Dragon Spiraling up the Pillar

This movement benefits the kidneys to nourish and support the heart and stimulates the cerebral spinal fluid, which bathes the brain and spine.

1. Stand with your feet together or slightly apart if you have difficulty with balance.
Inhale
2. As you keep your torso upright, bend your knees and lower your body down, keeping your arms at your sides.
Exhale
3. Twist your upper body to the right, looking back over your right shoulder; slowly straighten your knees as you turn.
4. Simultaneously swing your arms so your left forearm rests across your chest and your left hand on your right shoulder; at the same time place your right hand on your midback (or lower back if you can't reach) with the back of your hand against your body.
Inhale
5. Bend your knees and come back to center, slowly unraveling your arms until they are by your sides.
Exhale
6. Spiral to the left: straighten your legs as you turn to gaze over your left shoulder. Your arm and hand placements will be reversed. This time your right hand and arm fold over your chest, with your right hand resting by the left shoulder, and your left arm reaching up the

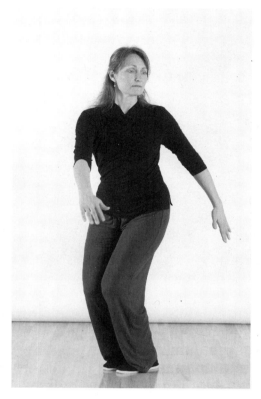

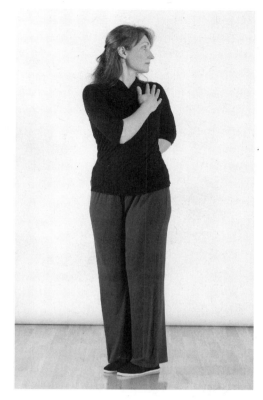

[17.1]

[17.2]

midback with palm facing outward. (See figs. 17.1 and 17.2.)

7. Inhale to center and continue spiraling back and forth. Repeat this exercise nine to eighteen times in each direction.

After you've become comfortable with this movement, add an extra step to the process. Pull in and up on your anus, vagina, and lower abdomen as you twist. This action helps to raise prolapsed organs and strengthen the bladder muscles to prevent incontinence.

Heart Healing Sound

The Six Healing Sounds are very effective if done at night to dispel toxins and emotions from the day, allowing surrender into deeper rest. Begin with the healing sound for the heart, performing this exercise six times, and then rest with a few *dantian* breaths. Do one to two more sets of six. (For a detailed description turn to chapter 8, Six Healing Sounds, p. 55.) You may also add any other healing sounds, depending on your condition or overriding emotion.

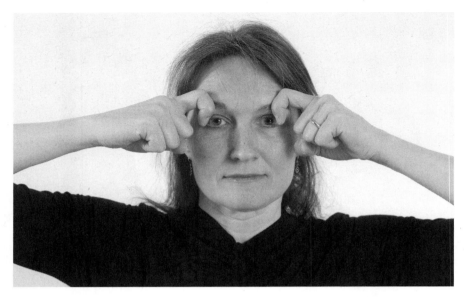

[17.3]

- For worrying, overthinking, or analyzing, add the Spleen Healing Sound.
- For anger, depression, a lot of dreams, or waking between 1:00 and 3:00 A.M., add the Liver Healing Sound.
- For night sweats and anxiety, include the Kidney Healing Sound.

STANCE

Three-Circles Stance

Do this stance during the day to build your immune system and the Three Treasures. Maintain the posture one to three minutes and work up to ten minutes or longer. (Turn to chapter 5, Stances, p. 31, for a full description.)

SELF-HEALING MASSAGE

Eyebrow Massage

Sit and rest your elbows on your chest so your head is relaxed and supported. Curl your index fingers into "C" shapes and place them on your inner eyebrows by the bridge of your nose. Massage along the eyebrows toward the temples for about two to three minutes or until you feel comfortable and relaxed. (See fig. 17.3.)

Neck Squeeze

Grab the back of your neck with one palm. Relax your hand as you take a deep breath. Exhale and squeeze out the tension from your neck muscles. You can sigh through your mouth for deeper relief. Continue for two minutes. At first your neck may be rigid but it will

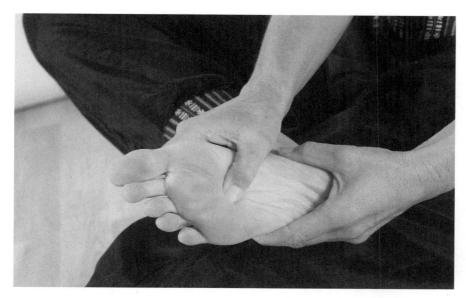

soften as you relax. This massage increases circulation (both Qi and blood) into the head and dispels tension in the neck.

Scalp Combing

Massage your scalp by combing your fingers through your hair to stimulate the acupuncture points on the head. Begin at the forehead and go back toward the base of the neck. Visualize releasing tension or negativity. Inhale to the top of the head and exhale to the neck, or exhale for the entire movement. Repeat twelve times.

Foot Massage

Before bed, soak in a footbath and massage Kidney 1, the acupuncture point in the middle of the upper third of the sole, in the center indentation when you squeeze your toes together. (See fig. 17.4.) Massaging this point will pull energy down from your head and help you relax. The kidney and heart are intricately connected, so working the feet helps settle the heart. If you have a willing partner, a foot massage in bed is really wonderful and relaxing. It puts me into a deep reverie.

MEDITATION

Buddha's Sleep

Assume this position while going to sleep or if you wake up in the middle of the night. Traditionally, Buddha's Sleep was thought to be the best posture for sleeping since the heart blood can circulate freely and the position of the intestines and stomach encourages the downward

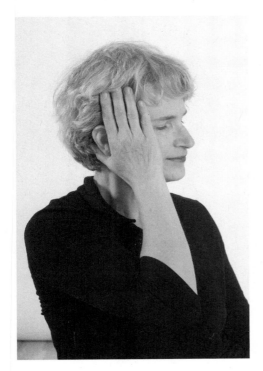

[17.5]

motion of digestion. The liver blood can also pool and be stored for the night. Lie and do deep *dantian* breathing. You can count your breaths or focus on the inhalation and exhalation until you fall asleep.

1. Place your right palm in front of your right ear (not covering) with your thumb below the earlobe and your fingers pointing toward your temple. (See fig. 17.5.) Lie down on your right side, keeping your hand in this position.

2. Lay your left hand on your left hip, with your legs comfortably bent. (You may want to place a pillow between your knees for comfort.)

3. Relax and concentrate on slow *dantian* breathing as you recline like the Buddha.

Practice the *Ren Chong* Meditation after your Qigong exercise routine and the Five-Eight Meditation before bed to help calm your nervous system. Descriptions for both of these meditations can be found in chapter 6, Meditations, on pp. 36 and 35, respectively.

ADDITIONAL HEALING AIDS AND CONTEMPLATIONS

Point Massage

Individually press and massage the wrist acupuncture points Pericardium 6 and Heart 7 for one to two minutes. You can stimulate these acupuncture points in bed, during your nighttime bath, or anytime during the day to relieve stress and anxiety.

Pericardium 6: This is the well-known point for alleviating motion sickness and upset stomachs. (There are bracelets to stimulate this point for relieving seasickness.) It has a calming affect on the emotions and body.

To locate P6, measure two thumb-widths up from your wrist crease on the inside (palm side) of your forearm. The point lies in the center between two tendons. Rub or press for a minute or longer.

Heart 7: This point is used for insomnia, heart palpitations, cardiac pain, and mental disorders. It's called *Shenmen* (*Shen* refers to spirit), so it's an important acupuncture point to calm your spirit and promote clarity.

This point can be found on the pinkie side of the wrist (on the ulnar side) at the wrist crease. If you splay your fingers, the point is on the medial side of the tendon that is palpable on the

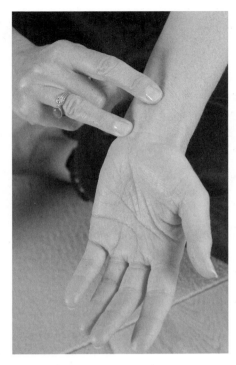

[17.6]

side of the wrist, although I've seen acupuncturists needle either side. Massage this area in small circles or hold the point to induce relaxation and to settle the heart. (See fig. 17.6.)

*Contemplations to Deepen
Your Healing*

- What are you taking into bed with you that you can leave behind or settle the following day?
- Are there recurring themes or life concerns that you need to address?
- Often women who have been sexually abused have insomnia. Make sure you feel

safe in your bedroom; place the bed in the proper feng shui position so you face the doorway.

A snoring partner can be very disruptive to your sleep. Before bed, have yours try nose oil (ayurvedic nasya oil is effective to moisten the sinus passages) and the nose strips available in drugstores. The last resort is to sleep separately so you can catch up on sleep. Don't let it go on for too long or you'll wear down your own body.

CONCLUSION

Insomnia has a variety of etiologies, but can be healed through Qigong, self-massage, meditation, and relaxation. I also prescribe herbal formulas, both Chinese and Western—patients with chronic, recalcitrant insomnia respond best when we alternate the herb formulas approximately every two to three weeks so the body doesn't get used to them. The Chinese formulas need to be prescribed by an acupuncturist or Chinese herbalist; however, the Western herbs such as passionflower, hops, chamomile, and lemon balm can be taken nightly as relaxing teas. I also use two dropperfuls of kava (a disgusting-tasting tincture) in soy milk or juice before bed to relieve anxiety-induced insomnia. Most of these herbs can be found in health food and herb stores along with a plethora of supplements. There are many remedies and programs to try, but the best cure for insomnia is a consistent Qigong practice to enable your body to reestablish its natural restful rhythms.

18

Breast Cancer and Other Types of Cancer

A wise man should consider that health is the greatest of human blessings, and learn how by his own thought to derive benefit from his illnesses.

—HIPPOCRATES

THE ETIOLOGY OF CANCER is complex and specific to each woman. In Chinese medicine, breast cancer is viewed as a progression of syndromes usually involving the liver and stomach meridians, which pass through the breasts bilaterally. Unexpressed or strong negative emotions, such as repressed anger and sorrow, are also contributing factors to cancer. The breast, a sensitive organ in women, is commonly a target.

Western medicine treats cancer like warfare, encouraging patients to hold the perception and imagery of "attacking the cancer" and "winning the battle" as a way to "be a survivor." The Qigong approach is quite different and focuses on cleansing toxins, balancing emotions, and strengthening immunity to counteract the cancer. Oriental therapy doesn't try to kill the "invaders" with drugs; rather, energy is focused on activating the healing power of the entire body. Cancer is considered an outcome of more severe and long-term disharmony of one's energy. Since the imbalance is internal, the individual (not the doctor or the drugs) holds the power of transformation and healing. Qigong is the key to activating the innate healer within and will stimulate the immune system and restore health no matter how weak a person has become.

Madame Guo Lin (1906–1984) was famous in China for healing herself from "incurable" uterine and bladder cancer with Qigong. She first underwent surgery for uterine cancer, which then reappeared and metastasized to her bladder. She was given six months to live. Unwilling to resign herself to death, she decided to explore the wisdom of Qigong that had been passed down through her Taoist family. With diligent practice, Guo Lin healed herself in six months.

Inspired by her miraculous results, she began teaching her Qigong cancer protocol, which became renowned throughout China. Guo Lin's Qigong focuses on walking and breathing routines to oxygenate the body and release toxins. These exercises have been successful for all types of cancer; many people have gone into remission while others report reduced pain and renewed vitality. Many practitioners and clinics worldwide have adopted her simple exercises as adjuncts to cancer treatment.

As long as you can breathe, you can heal yourself with Qigong. I have witnessed the power of Qigong to cure illnesses in many difficult cases where other doctors had given up and pronounced someone incurable.

One such person was Roberta.

She came to our Qigong clinic in Southern California with breast cancer that had metastasized throughout her body and had been told she only had three months to live—this after surviving an array of treatments, including numerous rounds of chemotherapy and radia-

tion. As with many people who came to our clinic, she was out of options and desperate for a cure.

In our approach to cancer, we always examine the emotions of the patient first, since they play an enormous role in both prevention and treatment of cancer (particularly breast cancer). In Roberta's case, she was extremely angry and distraught over her husband of twenty-eight years dumping her for a younger woman. Although it had been over five years since he had left, she was unwilling to let go of her resentment.

My Qigong teacher began his examination by asking poignant questions concerning her options and recommended that she examine her attitude toward her life and her family. He challenged her by asking: "How could you die and leave your ten-year-old daughter alone? Who will protect her and bring her up? You can't trust your husband to do it properly. You need to stay alive until your daughter reaches eighteen or twenty-one." Although this was an intimate commencement to her treatment, his honest approach served to boost Roberta's will to get better.

His next step was to reframe her divorce: he had her imagine that she had left her husband since he was unworthy of her love. "Change humiliation into renewed self-esteem," proposed Dr. Wu, knowing that a positive attitude is essential in healing. She still had a responsibility to live and needed to cultivate the mental stamina to make it through this ultimate challenge of life and death. Roberta's Qigong treatment involved reevaluating her perspective and lifestyle choices, to decide to move toward life and not death, which included following the Qigong program daily without fail.

With a death sentence looming over her, Roberta dedicated herself unequivocally to our program. During that year, she transformed her whole life by committing herself to incorporating Qigong and self-examination as the center of her new life. Not only did her tumors disappear, she emerged as a vibrant and passionate woman. We heard from her ten years later and she was still well, working two jobs to send her daughter to college!

In my clinic I prefer to create individualized programs for women based on a comprehensive Chinese medical diagnosis. Since women reading this book will be in different stages of their disease and recuperation, I've created a practice of fundamental Qigong exercises and meditations to launch them on their path to recovery, regardless of what type of cancer they have. During chemotherapy/radiation women usually get very weak and need to support their immune system and yin, both of which become deficient in these therapies. Acupuncture and herbs help tremendously, but it's imperative to do at least one breathing exercise daily—regardless of how weak you may feel. The more dedicated you are to your Qigong practice, the faster you will recover and regain your vitality.

MADAME GUO LIN'S CANCER EXERCISES

Then begin by performing *dantian* breathing throughout your day to gather energy and increase immunity, especially during drug treatments. You can do this in bed, in the clinic waiting room, or anytime you experience fearful thoughts. Simply focus your attention into your lower abdomen as you take long, deep, slow breaths. Just the breathing alone will help assuage fears and anxiety and promote a calm, positive attitude to activate your inner capacity to heal.

Remember: these exercises are beneficial for healing *all* types of cancers.

Guo Lin Walking

Walk outside, preferably in a quiet environment away from car exhaust and pollution. Surround yourself with trees, flowers, and beauty to infuse your cells with light and love, for optimal Qi healing. To get acquainted with the rhythm of this walk, imagine you are ice-skating, shifting your weight from side to side.

1. Inhale through your nose and exhale through your mouth for these exercises.
Inhale
2. Inhale through your nose while stepping forward to the right at a 45-degree angle.
3. Lift your left foot and briefly rest your left toes behind your right heel.
Exhale
4. Step with your left foot forward and to the side at a 45-degree angle.
5. Blow out twice through your mouth while stepping.
6. Briefly bring your right foot to rest behind your left heel, just before you take your next step.

7. Swing your arms like a pendulum as you walk, reaching both to the left and then to the right in rhythm with your breath. This increases the healing benefits of the movement. (See fig. 18.1.)

With each inhalation, visualize luminous Qi infusing each cell of your being, and then release the toxins on the exhalation. Walk for ten to twenty minutes at least once a day and more often if you can.

Alternative Breathing

As you feel stronger, switch to inhaling twice (as you step to one side) to increase your energy and exhaling once (to the other side). This is beneficial for walking up hills and will build your stamina.

When you're feeling weaker, with more symptoms present, focus on exhaling to expel the pathogens from your body and to move stagnant energy. Step and inhale once through the nose; on the next step blow two to three breaths out through your mouth.

It doesn't matter which side you choose to begin on—you can inhale to either side. Remember to coordinate your breathing with your steps. If you exhale (or inhale) twice, that is synchronized with one step. The ratio of inhalations to exhalations depends on your intention and condition: multiple inhalations increase your stamina while the exhalations detoxify the body more.

Rocking Breath

Imagine a horizontal line in front of you and place your feet on either side of the line—with the heel of one foot and the toes of the other foot on the line. Your feet should be hip- or shoulder-width apart. Stretch your arms overhead with your fingers interlaced, or raise one arm overhead and keep one by your side. Holding your arms upward improves lymphatic drainage in the chest.

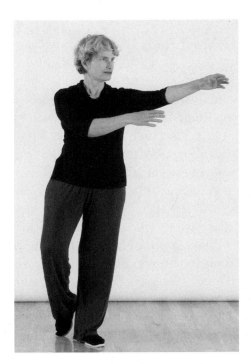

[18.1]

1. Rock back and forth on your feet.
2. Push forward on the inhalation while lifting your back heel and shifting your weight to your front foot. (See fig. 18.2.)
3. Press backward on the exhalation, lifting the toes of your front foot.

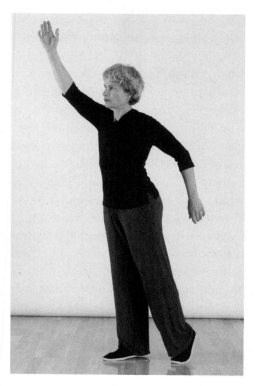

[18.2]

4. Inhale twice through your nose as you lean forward and blow out twice through your mouth as you rock back.

Continue two to three minutes and then switch feet.

STANCES

Three-Circles Stance

Perform this stance if you're strong enough (see page 31 in chapter 5, Stances). This will increase your immune power and is the most effective Qigong stance to gain strength. Begin

with one minute twice a day and slowly increase the time.

SELF-HEALING MASSAGE

Very Important Note: I don't prescribe massage with breast cancer because of the possibility of spreading the disease; this includes not massaging your healthy breast either. Instead, massage your feet, particularly the area above your small toes on the top (dorsal) part of both feet. This spot corresponds to your breasts in foot reflexology and will stimulate lymph drainage in the chest.

MEDITATIONS AND VISUALIZATIONS

Buddha's Sleep

This simple breathing builds immunity even if your condition is debilitating and all you can do is lie in bed. I've taught Buddha's Sleep to numerous cancer and AIDS patients who relied on this posture to sustain their energy and strength while bedridden.

1. Place your right palm in front of your right ear (not covering) with your thumb below the earlobe and your fingers pointing toward your temple. (See fig. 18.3.)Lie down on your right side, keeping your hand in this position.

2. Lay your left hand on your left hip, with your legs comfortably bent. (You may want to place a pillow between your knees to help promote relaxation and comfort.)

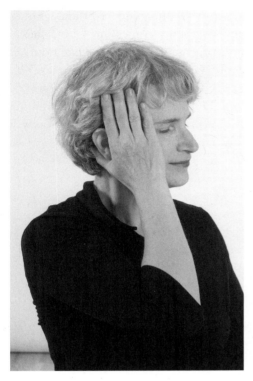

[18.3]

3. Concentrate on doing deep *dantian* breathing as you recline like the Buddha.

Begin with five minutes and increase to twenty. This will help fortify your immune system and cultivate Qi in the *dantian*. If you're too weak to get up, this is a good way to spend the time in bed!

Ren Chong *Meditation*

Ren and *chong,* the two important meridians for women's health, distribute Qi and blood into the chest region to enhance healing. Perform this meditation for ten minutes after your Qi-gong exercises to gather the healing Qi into your breasts and chest. For a more detailed description of this meditation, turn to chapter 6, Meditations, p. 36.

Sitting Forgetfulness

Relax into a comfortable meditation posture or lie down. Take ten deep, slow breaths and let go of any tension. Then follow your breath, watching it flow in and out of your body. Allow thoughts to float by, without focusing on them. After a while forget about your breath and your body and merge with the healing and expansive energies of the Universe. Sit for ten to twenty minutes or more.

Contemplations to Deepen Your Healing

- How are you nurturing and supporting yourself now? Do you nurture others more than yourself?
- Dialogue with your breast in a journal to express all of your feelings about the disease and loss.
- If your life were a story and breast cancer (or any other cancer) came in the form of a guide or teacher, what would that guide or teacher tell you? How would the story end?
- How has your inner landscape changed since getting breast cancer? How can you learn to be with this new landscape?
- Perform a grief ritual to honor the loss of your breast(s). I've seen women make papier-mâché casts of their breasts before mastectomies and create rituals or art pieces, inviting close women friends to be

present to witness and support their healing process.

CONCLUSION

To heal from all forms of cancer (including breast cancer) it's best to perform Qigong throughout the day. You can do one-half to one full hour in the morning and then again in the afternoon. Some clinics in China have the patients practicing Qigong for five hours a day. Madame Guo Lin reportedly practiced two hours every morning to initiate her remarkable healing. Don't strain, but do try to maintain a consistent practice to support your body in its healing process.

19

Heart Health
and Hypertension

*Love is the threshold where divine and human presence
ebb and flow into each other.*

—John O'Donohue

In Chinese medicine the intricate balance of mind, body, and spirit is controlled by the heart as well as the circulation of blood, patency of the vessels, and our overall health. The heart is not regarded solely as an organ; rather, it is considered something greater, a chamber that houses our consciousness and oversees the activities of our mind: keen thinking, memory, sleep, and our spiritual connection to life.

According to Chinese pathology, a major cause of heart disease is the lack of Qi, which supplies the energy to move the blood through the heart and vessels. Qi and blood are intricately related and heart disease is considered a progressive imbalance of these two synergistic elements. The heart symptom of pain radiating down the arm (known in Western medicine as referred pain) is actually signaling an energy imbalance along the heart meridian. A typical disease pattern may develop as follows: insufficient Qi decreases the blood flow to the heart, which in turn creates Qi and blood stagnation. This accumulation leads to blocked arteries and weakened heart function, and can eventually result in a heart attack or stroke from severe blood stasis.

Qigong is an important adjunct to treating heart disease because it builds people's energy and regulates their heart naturally. Through deep abdominal breathing and gentle movements to activate the heart and associated meridians, you can build your energy reserves and direct the Qi to the heart, strengthening and calming the cardiac and nervous systems. Please consult your physician before beginning any new exercise program, especially if you have heart issues.

EMOTIONS OF THE HEART

The heart is considered the "Supreme Ruler" and must be protected to live a long life. In the West we often consider the heart as the source of our feelings and emotions, so it would come as no surprise to learn that emotions do affect our cardiac health. When the heart's energy is imbalanced by anxiety, the mind becomes restless at night, producing insomnia, excess dreaming, and forgetfulness. Physical weakness and fatigue can also create symptoms such as depression, anxiety, heart palpitations, poor memory, and irregular heartbeats. One may sink into low spirits and appear lackluster, devoid of "fire" and passion.

Joy is essential in maintaining cardiovascular health. In my practice, I've seen many people who have "closed their hearts," not allowing love into their lives, afraid of intimacy and vulnerability. Some have lost someone dear to them and have locked that pain inside, or others were hurt as children and still carry the wounds as adults. These unhealed emotions and pain determine the level of our well-being, and if ignored, can lead to heart and other health conditions.

An important heart remedy is meditation. Many spiritual practices focus on opening the heart and cultivating compassion for ourselves, our families, our communities, and the world. This helps us keep a broader perspective on what's really important in our life. And, of course, laughter *is* the best medicine. Studies show that laughter lowers blood pressure and relieves stress; so relax, spend time with friends and loved ones, and enjoy life.

During my apprenticeship I was thrust into a life-threatening situation with a heart patient —my mother. One Sunday afternoon my mother and I were reading on the porch when all of sudden she became pale and clammy. The next moment she was bent over in her chair. As a budding acupuncture student, instead of calling 911, I immediately dug my fingernail into the acupuncture "emergency point" right above her upper lip. (I don't advise that you try this until after you call 911 *first* to make sure the person receives the best emergency care available, for their safety.) Within seconds, she began to recover; color returned to her face and she slowly stabilized. It might sound odd for me to take such a risk, but I really wanted proof that acupuncture works. I then drove her to the hospital where the physician recommended that she increase her cardiac medication and rest.

In the upcoming days, the prescription made her blood pressure spike dangerously high, along with causing frequent bouts of dizziness and arrhythmia. Frightened by her body's reaction to the drugs, she agreed to try some of the healing exercises I was learning from my Qigong instructor. Over the years my mother had volunteered to try many of my alternative healing experiments—taking herbal concoctions and other "weird" remedies. So she was open to try one more "experiment" that I believed would benefit her more than her prescribed drugs.

I designed a daily Qigong program for her heart (described in this chapter), which she practiced for fifteen minutes, twice a day. After following the Qigong routine for one month, I received an ecstatic call: "Deb, my pressure is down to 105/86! It hasn't been this low since I was in my twenties. I can't believe it!" Her cardiologist was baffled since she had decreased (rather than increased as he had recommended) her medications. Unfortunately, she didn't share that the secret of her improvement was Qigong! Later my mother sheepishly admitted that she was too restless to meditate but loved the exercises and followed them faithfully.

This Qigong combination of active and quieting exercises will regulate the heart and help soften and dilate blood vessels. While performing Qigong, focus on letting go of stress and anxiety with each exhalation. On the inhalation, breathe in peacefulness and imagine your heart expanding to embrace comforting and loving energy. You can even bathe your heart in red, the healing hue of the heart. Attune to your inner rhythm as your blood circulates and nourishes your entire body.

DYNAMIC EXERCISES AND HEALING SOUNDS

These exercises can be used for a variety of heart conditions, such as coronary heart disease, hypertension, anxiety disorders, stress, palpitations, irregular heart rhythms, and insomnia.

Remember: It is imperative that you consult your doctor or health care practitioner before starting any new exercise program.

Heart's Gentle Rock

This exercise is effective for lowering high blood pressure and increasing circulation in your legs. Often heart patients experience poor circulation and get edema in the ankles, so this is an important exercise to gently pump the blood from the legs back toward the heart. This is also a valuable exercise for people suffering from varicose veins and is suitable for women in a weakened state.

1. Stand in Basic Qigong Stance.
Inhale
2. Close your hands into loose fists. Raise them up to your sides so they are resting next to your ribs. Bend your elbows at right angles, with your palms facing up.
3. Simultaneously lift your left leg so your thigh is parallel to the ground. (See fig. 19.1.)
Exhale
4. Step forward with your left leg and place your heel on the floor. Slowly rock forward so you are shifting your weight to the front of your foot. Keep your right foot on the ground, without lifting up the heel.
5. At the same time, press out with open palms, extending your arms out in front of your body, with your palms facing away from you at heart level. (See fig. 19.2.)
Inhale
6. Slowly bring your arms back to your sides into a fist position. Rock back on your left heel and flex your left foot by lifting your toes. Your

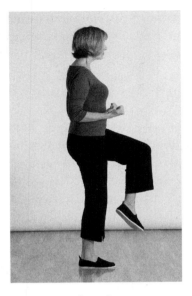

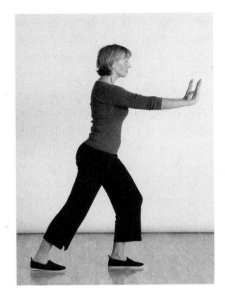

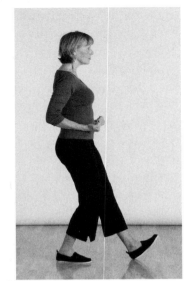

[19.1]   [19.2]   [19.3]

right knee should be bent and bearing most of your weight. (See fig. 19.3.)

7. Repeat this rocking motion while gently pushing forward and pulling backward.

8. Perform this nine times and then change legs.

9. Lift your right knee and step out with your heel and continue rocking nine times on this side. Repeat in increments of nine.

Gradually build up your stamina so you can do up to sixty-four repetitions on each side, but be sure you don't tire yourself out. This should be a relaxing and calming movement.

Floating Crane

This gentle Qigong stimulates circulation and is suitable for older or weaker women.

1. Stand in Basic Qigong Stance. Extend your arms out in front of your body, holding them at shoulder level, your palms facing down.

2. Press your arms up and down using a slight waving motion as you move your body up and down by slightly bending your knees. (You can stand and wave your arms, if bending is too strenuous in the beginning.)

Continue for one to five minutes. Be sure you do not overstrain in any of the heart exercises.

Heart Healing Sound

This exercise relieves stress, calms palpitations, and is helpful in maintaining overall cardiac health. Since the Six Healing Sounds detoxify the system of toxins and unwanted emotions gathered during the day, the exhalation is prolonged. A detailed description of this Qigong exercise can be found in chapter 8, Six Healing Sounds p. 55.

STANCES

Eagle Drying Her Wings

This stance will promote Qi and blood circulation, especially to your heart.

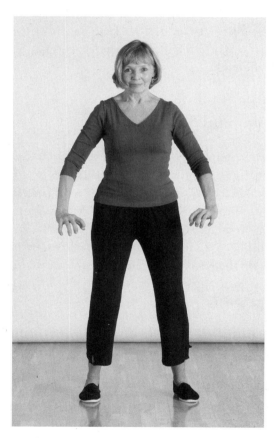

[19.4]

1. Stand with your knees comfortably bent; slightly lift the elbows away from your body out to the sides, as if you're holding a small ball under each armpit.

2. Bend your fingers as if grasping the lid of a jar. (See fig. 19.4.)

Hold for 1–5 minutes and practice abdominal breathing. Repeat one to two times a day.

SELF-HEALING MASSAGE

Self-massage is an integral part of Heart Qigong, to help stimulate the circulation and to redirect disruptive energy downward away from the heart. Most people find it is easier and more comforting to rub their bellies while lying in bed in the morning or in the evening before sleep. It is best to massage yourself on an empty stomach or wait at least an hour after a meal.

Ren Mai *Massage*

This massage is especially beneficial for palpitations, anxiety, and insomnia. Massage your torso nine times, moving from your diaphragm to your pubic bone (see chapter 13, PMS, p. 96 for description).

Eye Bath

1. Rub your hands together vigorously until your palms are warm.

2. Place your palms over your eyes, take a few deep breaths, and relax deeply.

This is especially soothing for stress or eye-strain and can be done anytime during the day.

MEDITATION

Meditation is the first step in regulating the heart and is one of the most important practices for healing any cardiac condition. Five-Eight Meditation will help you relax and remain calm, avoiding reactivity and stress, which weaken heart Qi. Sit for ten to twenty minutes. (For a more thorough discussion about Five-Eight Meditation, please read chapter 6, Meditation, on p. 35.)

HYPERTENSION (HIGH BLOOD PRESSURE)

Qigong can regulate blood pressure without medication, but if you are on medication it's advisable to have your doctor monitor your changes as you progress in your practice. My Chinese teacher loved to play tricks on American doctors and could alter his pressure at will by doing Qigong. Once during an annual physical, he raised his blood pressure just for fun, alarming the nurses. Then he sat in the examination room and lowered it on the spot, further confounding the medical staff. Of course, he's practiced Qigong cultivation for years, but this illustrates the potential power of our mind-body connection.

Hypertension has different causative factors, usually involving the kidney, liver, and heart meridians. One common syndrome is described in the metaphorical imagery of the Five Elements, where the Water (kidney, the mother of the liver) is not sufficient to nourish the Wood (liver), resulting in a flare-up of heat affecting the heart (see chapter 7, Five-Element Healing, p. 47). Stress, pent-up emotions, and overwork will affect blood pressure. I hear many stories where patients' hypertension was under control for years until they were faced with an IRS audit, or a personal trauma that immediately spiked their numbers. It's important to eliminate stressors and adopt new patterns of behavior and thinking that will bring balance and an enhanced ability to respond to challenges.

DYNAMIC EXERCISES

In the same way that my mother's practice of Qigong strengthened her heart, the protocol also helped to reduce her high blood pressure. Within a month of following her new routine, her blood pressure was under control. For a complete Qigong hypertension routine, be sure to add the Kidney and Liver Healing Sounds to your heart program, along with the following suggestions.

Bear Stretching

1. Stand in Basic Qigong Stance, or slightly wider to maintain balance.

Inhale

2. Bring your fists to your waist, palm-side up.

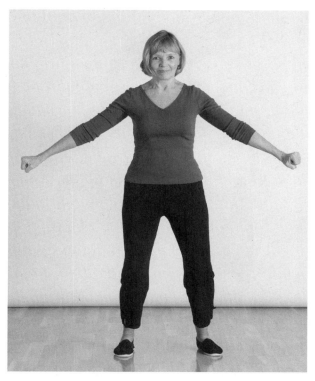

[19.5]

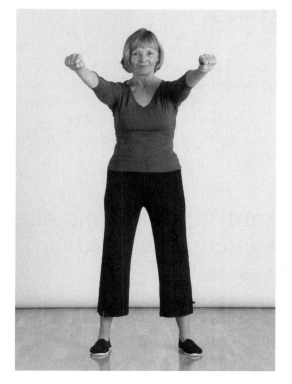

[19.6]

Exhale

3. Squat down as you punch your arms out to the side (as though you are hitting someone in the groin). (See fig. 19.5.)

Inhale

4. Bring your arms back to your waist with palms facing upward, as before. Remain in a squatted position.

Exhale

5. Next, stand up and simultaneously punch forward in a 45-degree angle at chin level (forming a "V" with your arms). (See fig. 19.6.)

Complete eight rounds. This was traditionally done in four directions (both clockwise and counterclockwise), turning your body to face each direction for the entire sequence.

Backward Walk or Run

This is a great way to improve your balance and coordination. Sometimes people will incur a stroke from high blood pressure. In walking or running backward, more motion tracks are created in the brain to aid in stroke prevention and recovery (see chapter 11, Wise Woman, p. 81 for details).

STANCE

The Three-Circles Stance or Hugging the Tree Pose are particularly helpful for hypertension and heart conditions (turn to chapter 5, Stances, pp. 31 and 30 respectively). By holding your arms at heart level, Qi and blood flow are stimulated in the chest, which helps regulate heart function.

ADDITIONAL HEALING AIDS AND CONTEMPLATIONS

Acupressure

Acupressure is an integral component of Qigong healing, and is a valuable aid when disturbing symptoms arise. One of the pressure points I taught my mother was to squeeze the tip of her left pinkie (acupuncture point Heart 9) when she felt heart symptoms coming on. This will regulate the heart instantly. Recently I witnessed the positive effects of this potent point when my mother was in intensive care recovering from surgery. She was experiencing atrial fibrillations (when the heart beats irregularly and rapidly), which the doctors were unable to regulate. Whenever she pressed Heart 9 or practiced deep abdominal breathing, her heart would immediately calm down; in fact, as I watched the monitors above her bed, I could see her rhythms become regular. It was fascinating to receive instant feedback recording the powerful effects of simple Qigong breathing and acupressure amid the chaos of intensive care.

Another valuable point is Governing Vessel

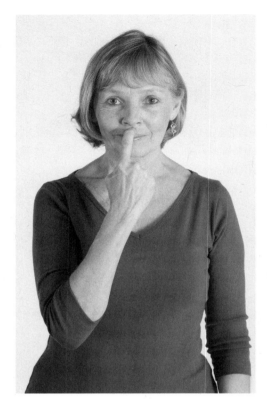

[19.7]

26—the point I pressed to revive my mother before driving her to the hospital. GV 26 is called a "revival point" in acupuncture because it can bring someone out of unconsciousness immediately. It is also used to relieve acute back sprain. I teach this to nurses, teachers, and health care practitioners whenever I have the opportunity. Everyone should know this important point since it can save lives.

GV26 is located midway along the vertical groove between the nose and upper lip. In an emergency, call 911 immediately and then attend to the person by digging your nail into this point or using the eraser side of a pencil to press hard. Remember, since they are unconscious, they will not feel your nail—but if they do, you're doing it right! (See fig. 19.7.) Of course these days there are probably liability issues in helping a stranger, but it's invaluable information to know and use for your family and friends.

Contemplations to Deepen Your Healing

- How are you receiving and giving joy?
- What pressures or concerns can you "lift off your chest" to allow more ease in your daily life?
- What emotions are you not venting that are building up inside?

- When was the last time you felt ecstatic joy? Imagine that now and feel it pulse through your body.
- Which projects have gone uncompleted because of depression or procrastination?
- What "fires you up" in life?

CONCLUSION

A daily Qigong practice can literally save your life. You can learn to naturally lower blood pressure, harmonize your heart rhythm, and increase Qi and blood circulation for a healthier heart. Qigong strengthens and regulates your cardiac and nervous systems and increases your physical and emotional stamina.

20

Osteoporosis

Walk around feeling like a leaf. Know you could tumble any second.
Then decide what to do with your time.

— Naomi Shihab Nye

The onset of Osteoporosis is usually associated with menopause; however, it has recently been discovered that our bones actually begin to lose their peak mass in our late thirties. This is a silent occurrence where the devastating effects of bone deterioration aren't perceived until we reach our seventies, often when it's too late to reverse the process. Therefore, it is essential to regard your bones as the inner foundation of your body, supporting you throughout your life with strength and resilience. In my travels to various countries I observed that older women in indigenous cultures did not get osteoporosis or the degenerative diseases that plague Western women. They were physically active, carrying heavy loads well into their elder years with ease and

grace. These women exuded an intimate connection to the Earth, rooted like ancient trees with a strong sense of their bodies and their place in the community.

The two factors I gleaned from observing these women were the importance of movement and their participation in weight-bearing activities. Women who don't exercise are more prone to osteoporosis since exercise stimulates the bones to absorb calcium and remain strong. As we age, according to Chinese medical theory, our kidney energy wanes, compromising our bone formation and health. In addition, the spleen's ability to absorb nutrients is not as robust as in our youth, so our ability to utilize key minerals (like calcium) and nutrients from our food is often impaired.

Socially and culturally, there is a lot of fear around growing old or aging in general, and women are especially prone to this fear as they enter menopause. The emotion of fear further weakens the kidney Qi. Healing must include facing your fears and examining your beliefs about aging, as well as remaining active.

When women are in perimenopause, I suggest that those who have osteoporosis in their family include a bone scan as part of their medical checkup to determine the baseline of their bone density. One of my patients, Susan, was forty-seven when she came to my clinic with moderate osteoporosis that she discovered with a heel test performed at her health club. Fearful of the inevitable deterioration and frailty that her physician described, she was anxious to take the prescribed osteoporosis drug, but I convinced her to try Qigong first for three to six months to see how her bones responded.

She had not exercised much in her life, so initially she tired easily and was only able to exercise for about twenty minutes a day. But as she continued her new program of Qigong and walking (practiced in short sessions throughout the day), by the end of six months she was hiking for hours each day and was able to stand on one foot to perform the Qigong Crane Series. (This series is a more advanced form of Qigong that requires balancing on one foot while stretching in different balancing poses.) This focused weight-bearing exercise promotes long bone formation, strengthens tendons and ligaments, and increases coordination and balance. Within six months her bone density was better than normal and she had become fit and strong in the process. I've also recommended the Eight-Brocade and kidney exercises described in this chapter with equal success, a series of exercises that are more suitable for older women.

DYNAMIC EXERCISES

This Qigong program tones the kidneys and emphasizes stimulation of the long bones, which are prone to deterioration. Add these exercises to your daily Qigong routine if you're a menopausal or postmenopausal woman. You can perform these exercises for prevention of or to heal osteoporosis.

Shoulder Shrugging

This is the *best* exercise for osteoporosis. The jarring on the heels stimulates the brain to send calcium to the long bones to build more bone mass and promote strength. (For a full description of this turn to chapter 4, Activating Your Energy, p. 24.) You can practice Shoulder Shrugging once or twice a day.

One-Foot Thud

Substitute this exercise if you find Shoulder Shrugging too strenuous or uncomfortable on your feet. Turn to chapter 12, Sage Woman, p. 84 for a full description.

Eight-Brocade Kidney Posture

1. Stand in Basic Qigong Stance.
Inhale

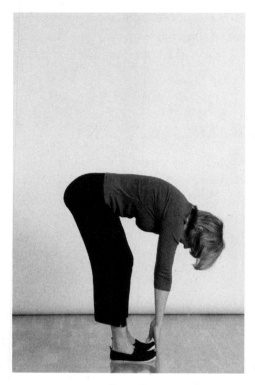

[20.1]

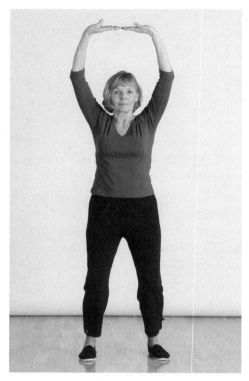

[20.2]

2. No movement.

Exhale

3. Bend forward from your waist and grasp your toes with your fingers, touching the acupuncture point Bubbling Spring (Kidney 1), which can be found in the middle of the ball of your foot.

Inhale

4. Relax slightly as you remain in this position.

Exhale

5. Pull your toes toward your head, keeping your arms straight as you round your back up-

ward, forming an elongated oval. If you can't reach your toes, just lift them toward you as you bend. Focus on creating a stretch in your middle and lower back as you pull on your toes. (See fig. 20.1.)

6. Hold your head up, look slightly forward, but don't strain your neck.

Relax on the inhalation and stretch your back up as you exhale. Repeat three times. Feel the energy connecting between the balls of your feet and the kidneys in your back. You can feel the energy circulating in your whole body once you become acquainted with the movement.

Pillar Holding the Heavens

1. Stand in Basic Qigong Stance.
Inhale
2. Raise your palms in front to your chest with palms facing upward, fingers pointing toward each other.
3. Simultaneously bend your knees (as you bring your hands up to chest level).
Exhale
4. Rotate your hands outward until your palms are facing skyward with the fingers still close together.
5. Press the palms upward, stretching your arms overhead, like you're a pillar, holding the heavens.
6. Concurrently straighten your legs as you push your hands above your head. Keep your head level as you look forward. (See fig. 20.2.)

Feel the strength of your body, with your feet planted into the Earth, your whole body dynamic and solid. Hold your breath for a few moments to augment the sense of power. Repeat three times.

STANCE

Three-Circles Stance

This posture will help to strengthen your legs and thighs. As you stand in Modified Horse Stance, be sure that your knees don't extend over your toes. Hold for three to ten minutes (see chapter 5, Stances, p. 31).

SELF-HEALING MASSAGE

Massage your kidney area frequently with your palms or loose fists until your back is warm. Since the kidneys promote bone growth, send healing Qi into the kidneys as you stimulate and warm them.

MEDITATION

Mindfulness Meditation is always helpful to calm the mind and settle the whole body into deeper relaxation. You may finish your meditation by sending healing light into your bones, visualizing their growth, strength, and stability. (See chapter 6, Meditations, p. 34.)

ADDITIONAL HEALING AIDS

Hiking is an effective weight-bearing exercise that will complement your Qigong. Carry a daypack with some weight to stimulate bone strength and growth, and if you're fit you can add twenty to thirty pounds to augment the weight-bearing effect. Also, jumping exercises are beneficial for bone formation.

The Chinese favor soups with tendons, cartilage, and bones to build their skeletal systems.

Tofu and soybeans may be more palatable additions to your diet for hormonal and bone nourishment. One of my acupuncture teachers ate sardines, dry-fried in a pan with sliced almonds, flavored with tamari and maple syrup. It's actually a very tasty and nutritious snack. Eat protein to build your bones, and take in plenty of dark green, leafy vegetables. Try to refrain from the following activities since they compromise bone health: smoking, drinking sodas, an excessive intake of alcohol and caffeine, and too much exercise.

Dr. Wu is also adamant about proper anatomical alignment while doing your workout. Using treadmills and other exercise machines can create malpositioning of the bones and cause undue stress on the musculoskeletal system. Notice how people work out on machines and you'll be surprised at how torqued their bodies appear as they exercise. Become more aware of your body in space and how you carry yourself throughout your daily activities.

CONCLUSION

Begin to take care of your bones today. Get up and move and initiate some changes in your daily routines. Walk up stairs instead of taking the escalators, park farther away from the store and carry your groceries to strengthen your arms. Eat and exercise in moderation, since too little or too much of either is detrimental to skeletal health. Qigong will empower you with the ability to keep yourself strong, standing tall, and anchored like an oak tree.

21

Restoring Your Sexual Qi

I want to do with you what spring does with the cherry trees.

—Pablo Neruda

It's natural for a woman's sexual energy to flow in cycles, sometimes juicy and inviting, other moments quiet and inward. These rhythms fluctuate during our life, coinciding with our age and where we are in our life's journey. Right before the reproductive capacity wanes, women often enjoy a peak of sexual activity in their early forties. Then they may experience a decline in interest with the onset of menopause, although I have met women who blossom sexually once they're liberated from becoming pregnant. Apart from hormones, our attitude definitely influences how we perceive and experience our sensuality as we age.

During midlife the kidney energy, which sustains our reproductive organs and sexual drive, is diminishing. The nourishing waters of the body (yin) begin to dissipate and symptoms of heat and dryness ensue, such as waning vaginal fluids, hot flashes, night sweats, and dry skin. But even with this natural decline, we can keep our sexual lives vibrant by focusing on toning (nourishing) the kidneys and bringing renewed energy to the pelvis and genitals. As you concentrate your cultivated Qi into the Uterine Palace through these Qigong exercises, your natural desire for sex will reawaken and lovemaking will become more enjoyable.

When I was in acupuncture school, I had long days of classes and clinical internships. All of my energy went into studying and I had lost my desire for sex. One day my Qigong master said, "Oh, Deborah, you're too young to not have sexual feelings. This means your kidneys need some warming energy to restore their yang Qi." I lay down on my stomach and he placed his hands about a foot above my lower back. Instantly I felt warm liquid energy streaming into my kidney area. His Qi treatment lasted about ten minutes. I felt warm and comfortable, but not sexual in that moment. He then taught me the exercises that follow to increase my libido and sustain the energy that he'd transmitted to my kidneys.

That weekend I went to a party and felt like a wild bull on the run. My sexuality was overflowing and I could hardly maintain my composure. I wanted to make love and wasn't going home without a man! Luckily everyone was paired up at the party so I was saved from myself, but the Qigong reawakened my sexuality like a volcano about to explode. I returned to my teacher on Monday and asked him to turn it off before it got me into trouble!

In Chinese medicine, there is a theory that too much sex will diminish one's kidney energy. So he taught me how to gather the Qi and not squander the energy. It is also important to not have intercourse right after doing your Qigong practice so you can store the Qi garnered within your *dantian* and Uterine Palace. This experience during my apprenticeship convinced me unequivocally of the potency of Qigong and the tremendous potential for transforming our own energy. Even though it might seem easier to have a Qigong master around the house to rekindle your sexual Qi, you too can develop this capability within yourself.

To cultivate your sexual energy, add these exercises to your regular Qigong routine. I suggest performing your other exercises first and then directing the cultivated Qi into your kidneys and reproductive organs through the Sexual Qigong. These exercises require that your attention be more focused and internal, gathering energy into your Uterine Palace to energize your libido. These movements will increase kidney energy, harmonize your mind and body, increase pelvic Qi, and restore youthful vigor.

DYNAMIC EXERCISES

Coccyx Exercises

This Qigong will increase sexual libido by activating the Qi and yang circulation in the pelvis. They are subtle movements that require concentration on the micromovements of the coccyx.

1. Stand with your feet a little wider than shoulder-width apart, knees slightly bent. Look down to make sure that your knees do not extend over your toes. Your feet and coccyx (the "tail" at the base of the spine) should form a triangle.

2. The point at the apex of your head (acupuncture point Governing Vessel 20) and your perineum (the area between your vagina and anus) should be aligned, with your coccyx back a bit.

3. Take a few deep belly breaths and feel yourself connected to the Earth before you start.

4. Concentrate on moving your coccyx in small micromovements in the three directions described below. The action does not take place in the buttocks or sacrum; it is very subtle and should hardly be seen.

5. Relax the rest of your body with slow Qigong breathing. Slowly move your tailbone nine to thirty-six times in each direction:
   • Forward and backward
   • Lateral side to side
   • Circle in both directions

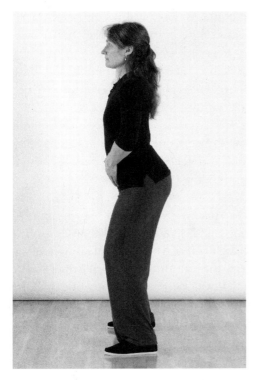

[21.1]

Pelvic Tilt

By focusing your breath into the Uterine Palace (see chapter 4, Activating Your Energy, p. 22, the Pelvic Tilt stimulates sexual energy and activates the Qi in the reproductive organs and pelvis.

1. Stand in Horse Stance (or the modified version). Be sure that your knees don't buckle inward or extend out over your toes.

2. Place one hand on your Uterine Palace (the area right above your pubic bone) and the other one on your sacrum (the triangular bone at the base of your spine).

Inhale

3. Slightly scoop your pelvis forward, pulling up gently on your perineum, vagina, and anus. Draw the energy into your Uterine Palace with your inhalation.

Exhale

4. Tilt your sacrum back and relax your pelvic floor, but keep some gentle tension present. (See fig. 21.1.)

5. As you continue scooping your pelvis back and forth, envision drawing a crescent moon or wiping the inside of a bowl with your pelvis.

Breathing slowly concentrates energy into the Uterine Palace. As you inhale, imagine your breath filling your Uterine Palace with healing and revitalizing Qi. This stimulates pelvic circulation and increases sensations in the genitals. This can be a very juicy movement! Repeat the pelvic tilt up to thirty-six times.

Pelvic Floor Lift

This exercise is good for increasing the energy in the reproductive organs and genitals, as well as energizing the Uterine Palace. (For a full description turn to chapter 16, Menopause, p. 117.)

STANCE

Practice the Awkward Stance (p. 31) for one to three minutes, slowly increasing the duration as you become stronger. This open-legged squat activates the three yin meridians (kidney, liver, and spleen) that run up the inside of the legs into the pelvis. They are particularly influential in a women's sexual health and vitality.

SELF-HEALING MASSAGE

Breast Massage

Massage your breasts quickly in small circles for thirty-six to one hundred times. Massaging the breasts stimulates sexual feelings and enhances pleasure in the body.

Ovary Breathing

This breath work concentrates the energy (Qi) into the Uterine Palace and will increase your libido. (See chapter 10, Graceful Passage, p. 74.)

ADDITIONAL HEALING AIDS

Kegels

Kegels are not a Qigong exercise, although the Chinese have their own version that has been used for centuries. Women insert polished jade eggs into their vaginas to exercise the vaginal and pelvic floor muscles. This technique helps strengthen the sexual organs, tones muscles after childbirth, increases Qi and blood circulation to the urinary and reproductive areas, and improves sexual pleasure and responsiveness.

Kegel exercises were developed by Dr. Kegel to prepare women for childbirth.

1. Squeeze your vaginal muscles for a slow count of ten.

2. Relax for a count of five and repeat.

3. Make sure your abdomen and buttocks remain relaxed and that you continue to breathe gently without holding your breath.

4. To check that you are using the right muscles, insert one or two fingers inside your vagina and feel the inner muscles squeezing around them.

Do this five times and repeat three times during the day. When you become comfortable with the exercise you can do it anywhere. I practice in the car or waiting in supermarket or postal lines. Be creative—no one will know! You can also buy plastic cones or glass or jade eggs to insert and hold in your vagina for a few minutes. These all create similar effects and come in various sizes and weights.

CONCLUSION

There are a plethora of Qigong exercises to increase your sexual energy and the Taoist masters are the most renowned for these practices. Much of the focus is on strengthening and invigorating the kidneys, including the Qi, yin, yang, and *Jing*, but it's also essential for a woman to concentrate her energies into her Uterine Palace and pelvic organs. Through these sexual Qigong movements you will learn to revitalize your Uterine Palace, ovaries, and reproductive energies to nourish the essence of your femininity. If you support this precious woman's energy center as you mature, you will have a nurturing and active sex life—regardless of your age.

ACKNOWLEDGMENTS

THIS BOOK HAS BEEN in gestation for so many years and has followed me through three different states and many transformations. I feel deep gratitude for all of my friends, colleagues, and guides, who supported me in this journey from the dolphin waters of Santa Barbara, through the sacred lands of Santa Fe, and on to the nurturing hills of Ashland, Oregon. Thanks and blessings for all of the people, named and unnamed, who held the vision for this manifestation.

To Ren: This book would have not been birthed without your knowledge and generosity. I am forever grateful for all of the years of teachings, intense trainings, Qi healings, care, and unconditional love. You have been my mentor, taskmaster, and friend, who always encouraged me despite my laziness. May you be released from all karma and be free!

To Daniel Lee: You were my anchor, my unwavering support, and the light in the depths of darkness. Thank you for your hugs, neck rubs, encouragement, emotional support, and of course your computer wizardry and graphic art. I can't thank you enough.

To Dr. Kevin Lee: I have great gratitude for your detailed illustrations that only a doctor could do! Thanks for your time, artistry, and focused intent, especially at the last moments of birthing this book.

To Gabrielle Leslie, my editor, who kept me focused and grounded, especially in the final hours: Thanks for midwifing this creation with me with grace and laughter.

To Steve Scholl: I'm so glad you took me under your wing before exiting the business. Thanks for holding my hand through the maze of publishing with your easygoing manner and smiles.

I am grateful to numerous friends who emotionally supported me in this journey: *Ted Baer,* the reluctant lawyer-poet, who encouraged me through the many incarnations of this book. Thanks for your laughter, wit, and friendship, and of course your lawyer advice and support. *Galen Buller,* my desert muse, thanks for supporting me in my newfound creativity with a gentle heart, yummy Santa Fe dinners, and the nuances of grammar. I also want to express appreciation to my other desert amiga, *Lindsay*

Robinson, for her care, open home, and cosmic crystal healings.

While writing this book, my mother passed away. I have deep gratitude for the women who cared for me in this difficult passage: *Charu Colorado,* you were my lifeline through my mother's death. Heartfelt thanks for keeping me together through your insightful dream wizardry and the insights from Byron Katie. *Debora Farrington,* thanks for your honesty, fiery spirit, and friendship through the years, especially through the bardo of mom's passage. *Lois Wagner,* you've been like a sister to me, so thoughtful and caring. I'm so glad you're part of my family.

To Beth Frankl and the Shambhala Staff: Thanks for believing in my vision and helping me birth my first book.

Many thanks to the people who helped with the book's production in Ashland, Oregon: *Robert Frost* for his professional photography, keen eye, and patience; *Rick Sultan* for his Zensho studio; *Nancy* at Dreamsacks for her luscious bamboo outfits; *Johanna Wright,* the beautiful Dynamic Woman; *Cathy Black,* the dancing, healing Wise Woman; *Marilyn Edwards,* the beautiful, dedicated Qigong Sage Woman; and *Susanne Petermann,* the poetic breast goddess, who also brought us polenta hearts at the final editing frenzy.

To ALL MY ANCESTORS, Spirits, the Immortals, and Kuan Yin, who guide me lovingly through this journey. I bow to all the directions in deep gratitude.

APPENDIX:
Summary of Qigong Routines

THE FOLLOWING IS a list of all of the programs described in this book—each routine contains the appropriate dynamic exercises, stances, self-healing massages, and meditations for each condition or age group.

DYNAMIC WOMAN SEQUENCE

Awkward Stance (p. 31): 3–10 minutes
Side Step (p. 64): 8 times each side
Beautiful Woman Pose (p. 66): 8 breaths
    each side
Snake Walk (p. 66): 16–32 times
Arm Wheel (p. 67): 64 times
Dunhuang Meditation (p. 36): 24 breaths
Ovary Bridge Massage (p. 68): 16 times or until
    warm
Ren Chong Meditation (p. 36): 10 minutes

GRACEFUL PASSAGE: PERIMENOPAUSE

Drinking Essence from Bubbling Spring
    (p. 71): 9–18 times

Flying Eagle (p. 72): 9–18 times
Snake Twist Walk (p. 73): 18–36 times
Awkward Stance or Three-Circles Stance
    (p. 31): 3–10 minutes
Large Intestine Massage (p. 74): 9–18 times
Ovary Breathing (p. 74): 8–64 times
Ren Chong Meditation (p. 36): 10 minutes

WISE WOMAN: AGES FIFTY
TO SIXTY-FOUR

Joint rotations (p. 76): 2–4 minutes
Four-Sided Knee Kick (p. 77): 4–8 rounds
Twisting Crane (p. 78): 9 times to each side
Crane Walk (p. 79): 1–3 minutes
Nourishing the Uterine Palace (p. 80): 24
    times
Dragon Spiraling up the Pillar (p. 122): 9–18
    times
Backward Walk or Run (p. 81): 50–200 steps
Three-Circles Stance (p. 31): 3–10 minutes
Kidney Massage (p. 81): 1–3 minutes
Five-Eight Meditation (p. 35): 5–15 minutes

SAGE WOMAN: SIXTY-FIVE AND BEYOND

Shoulder Shrugging or One-Foot Thud
     (pp. 24, 84): 1–3 minutes or 9–36 times
Side Hop (p. 84): 12 hops or 2 minutes
Figure Eight Walk (p. 85): 8 times each
     direction
Heart's Gentle Rock (p. 137): 9–18 times
Simple Snake Movements (p. 25): 9–18 times
Three-Circles Stance (p. 31): 1–5 minutes
Spiral Massage (p. 86): 24 out, 36 in
Five-Eight Meditation (p. 35): 10–20 minutes

PREMENSTRUAL SYNDROME (PMS)

Push the Mountain (p. 93): 9–18 times
Six Healing Sounds (pp. 53, 57): Liver and
     Spleen: 6 times for each organ
Soothing the Middle (p. 94): 18 times
Awkward Stance (p. 31): 3–10 minutes
Ren Mai Massage (p. 96): 18 times
Ren Chong Meditation (p. 36): 10 minutes

BREAST HEALTH

Lymph Pump (p. 100): 1 minute or longer
Six Healing Sounds (pp. 53, 57): Liver and
     Spleen: 6 times each
Happy Liver Stretch (p. 101): 9–18 times each
     side
Hugging the Tree Pose (p. 30): 3–10 minutes
Nurturing Earth Yin Breast Massage (p. 102):
     8 times both directions
Breast Snake Massage (p. 103): 3 times for each
     breast
Figure Eight Massage (p. 104): 8 times
Nipple Rebound (p. 104): 3 times

Breast Lift (p. 104): 32–48 times
Ren Chong Meditation (p. 36): 10 minutes

DEPRESSION

Whole-Body Pat (p. 24): 1–2 minutes
Body Shake (p. 109): 1 minute
Happy Liver Stretch (p. 101): 9–18 on each
     side
Snake (p. 109): 1 minute or longer
Push the Mountain (p. 93): 9–18 times
Six Healing Sounds: Spleen (p. 57), Liver
     (p. 53), Heart (p. 55): 6 times for each organ
Awkward Stance (p. 31): 1–3 minutes or
     longer
Liver 3 Massage (p. 111): 1–2 minutes
Floating Cloud Meditation (p. 111), or Sea
     Meditation (p. 35): 10–20 minutes

MENOPAUSE

Sweeping Water (p. 116): 9 times each
     direction
Push the Mountain (p. 93): 9–18 times
Pelvic Floor Lift (p. 117): 9–18 times
Six Healing Sounds (pp. 52, 56): Kidney and
     Triple Heater: 6 times for each
Awkward Stance (p. 31): 3–10 minutes
Ovary Massage (p. 118): 60–180 times
Dunhuang Meditation (p. 36): 5–10 minutes
Ren Chong Meditation (p. 36): 10 minutes
Mindfulness Meditation (p. 34): 10–20 minutes

INSOMNIA

Dragon Spiraling up the Pillar (p. 122): 9–18
     times each direction
Six Healing Sounds (p. 55): Heart: 6–12 times

Three-Circles Stance (p. 31): 3–10 minutes
Eyebrow Massage (p. 124): 2–3 minutes
Neck Squeeze (p. 124): 2 minutes
Scalp Combing (p. 125): 12 times
Foot Massage (p. 125): as long as you like
Buddha's Sleep (p. 125): as you go to sleep
Point Massage (p. 126): P6, Heart 7: 1–2
   minutes

BREAST CANCER AND OTHER TYPES OF CANCER

Guo Lin Walking (p. 130): 10–20 minutes
Rocking Breath (p. 131): 2–3 minutes each side
Three-Circles Stance (p. 31): 1–10 minutes
   each side
Buddha's Sleep (p. 132): 5–20 minutes
Ren Chong Meditation (p. 36): 10 minutes
Sitting Forgetfulness (p. 133): 10–20 minutes

HEART HEALTH

Heart's Gentle Rock (p. 137): 9–18 times each
   side
Floating Crane (p. 138): 1–5 minutes
Six Healing Sounds (p. 55): Heart: 6 times
Eagle Drying Her Wings (p. 139): 1–5 minutes
Ren Mai Massage (p. 96): 9 times

Eye Bath (p. 139): 1 minute
Five-Eight Meditation (p. 35): 10–20 minutes
(For Hypertension add)
Kidney/Liver Healing Sounds (pp. 52–53):
   6 times for each organ
Bear Stretching (p. 140): 8 times
Backward Walk or Run (p. 81): 50–100 steps

OSTEOPOROSIS

Shoulder Shrugging (p. 24): 1–3 minutes
One-Foot Thud (p. 84): 9–36 times each side
Eight-Brocade Kidney Posture (p. 145): 3 times
Pillar Holding the Heavens (p. 146): 3 times
Three-Circles Stance (p. 31): 3–10 minutes
Kidney Massage (p. 147): 1–3 minutes
Mindfulness Meditation (p. 34): 10–20 minutes

RESTORING SEXUAL QI

Coccyx Exercises (p. 150): 9–36 times each
   direction
Pelvic Tilt (p. 151): 9–36 times
Pelvic Floor Lift (p. 117): 9 times
Awkard Stance (p. 31): 3–10 minutes
Breast Massage (p. 152): 36–100 times
Ovary Breathing (p. 74): 8–64 times
Kegels (p. 152): 5 minutes

NOTES

CHAPTER 2. THE ENERGETIC BODY

1. Dianne Connelly, *Traditional Acupuncture: The Law of the Five Elements,* (Columbia, Md.: The Centre for Traditional Acupuncture, 1979), 34. This is a conversation between Ch'i Po, who was an acupuncture master, and the Yellow Emperor, from the ancient Chinese classic *Nei Ching.*
2. Shou-Yu Liang and Wen-Ching Wu, *Qigong Empowerment: A Guide to Medical Taoist Buddhist Wushu Energy Cultivation,* (East Providence, R.I.: The Way of the Dragon Publishing, 1997), 90.

CHAPTER 6. MEDITATIONS AND VISUALIZATIONS

1. Tulku Thondup, *The Healing Power of Mind,* (Boston, Mass.: Shambhala Publications, 1996), 41.
2. Thich Nhat Hanh, *Being Peace,* (Berkeley, Calif.: Parallax Press, 1987), 5.

CHAPTER 7. FIVE-ELEMENT HEALING

1. Thich Nhat Hanh, http://www.quotations page.com/quote/32069.html.

CHAPTER 15. DEPRESSION

1. Mary Oliver, "The Summer Day," *New and Selected Poems,* (Boston, Mass.: Beacon Press, 1992), 94.
2. Thomas Moore, *Care of the Soul: A Guide for Cultivating Depth and Sacredness in Everyday Life,* (New York: HarperCollins, 1992), 138, 146.

BIBLIOGRAPHY

Cleary, Thomas. *Immortal Sisters: Secret Teachings of Taoist Women*. Berkeley, Calif.: North Atlantic, 1989.

Cohen, Kenneth. *The Way of Qigong: The Art and Science of Chinese Energy Healing*. New York: Ballantine, 1997.

Connelly, Dianne. *Traditional Acupuncture: The Law of the Five Elements*. Columbia, Md.: The Centre for Traditional Acupuncture, 1979.

Haas, Elson. *Staying Healthy with the Seasons*. Berkeley, Calif.: Celestial Arts, 1981.

Kaptchuk, Ted J., OMD. *The Web That Has No Weaver: Understanding Chinese Medicine*. New York: Congdon & Weed, 1983.

Liangyue, Deng, et al. *Chinese Acupuncture and Moxibustion*. Beijing: Foreign Languages Press, 1987.

Low, Royston. *The Secondary Vessels of Acupuncture*. New York: Thorsons, 1983.

Maciocia, Giovanni. *The Foundations of Chinese Medicine*: *The Treatment of Diseases with Acupuncture and Chinese Herbs*. New York: Churchill Livingstone, 1989.

Northrup, Christiane, MD. *The Wisdom of Menopause: Creating Physical and Emotional Health and Healing During the Change*. New York: Bantam, 2001.

Oz, Mehmet, MD. *Healing from the Heart: A Leading Surgeon Combines Eastern and Western Traditions to Create the Medicine of the Future*. New York: Plume (Penguin Group), 1998.

Thondup, Tulku. *The Healing Power of Mind: Simple Meditation Exercises for Health, Well-Being, and Enlightenment*. Boston, Mass.: Shambhala, 1996.

Zhengcai, Liu. *The Mystery of Longevity*. Beijing: Foreign Languages Press, 1990.

PRODUCT
INFORMATION

IN THIS BOOK I REFER to my DVD, *The Spirit of Qi Gong: Chinese Exercises for Longevity*. It features guided routines of many of the exercises described here, such as the Six Healing Sounds for organ health. To order this DVD (also available in international video formats), as well as other books and DVDs, call 800-723-6966 or visit www.womensqigong.com.

A SCHEDULE OF WORKSHOPS and retreats, information about private consultations, and resources to help support your Qigong practice, can also be found on my Web site listed above.